Healing C[

Sexual Abuse:

An Art Therapist's Journey

By Ann Owen

outskirts
press

Endorsements

"Through original paintings and written reflections about this art and her personal experiences, Ann invites you into her world. It is a place of healing and spunky raw truths, a shared space in her heart. There, you are given ways to explore your own experiences by writing or making art, encouraged by Ann's ideas and open questions. This visual memoir of emotional and physical healing gives everyone permission to discover greater understanding of sexual abuse. Readers will see with fresh eyes through the stories Ann tells and the pastel images that go beyond words."

—Marjorie Isaacs, D. Psy

"Ann is what we might call a 'therapist's therapist.' In her powerful book *HEALING CHILDHOOD SEXUAL ABUSE* Ann gives us tools for discovering and resolving our own wounds and the wounds of others for whom we may serve as guides and counselors toward healing and wholeness. Ann Owen's wise and sensitive, heart-centered words and 'works of art' allow our bodies and minds to find respite and insight along the path to recovery. Brava, Ann! Thank you for your courage and artistic vision, love and gratitude."

—Dr. Rebecca A. Martin

"Ann's book is a guide so helpful to any victim of childhood sexual abuse. As a developmental psychologist, I have learned that young children have no way to conceptualize their abuse or abuser. Number 1, because often symbolic language is yet undeveloped, and Number 2—and more to the point—they have no knowledge of sexuality—nor should they! Abuse is experienced without words—abuse is experiences, stored and retrieved in emotions and imagery. Healing and health happens when you have the courage to be your own hero or heroine. Ann's book is a precious guide and touchstone; Ann clearly speaks your language. Lean on her. Once you do, you will find validation and the inner strength you ALWAYS had! Bless you, Ann, and bless you, reader!"

—Anne Conkin, M.Psy.

"Ann Owen presents the reader a process to uncover the hidden mysteries of the psyche. She is candid in uncovering and reporting to the reader her hidden depths. Her ability to find her truths gives the reader the hope and belief that they too may discover and release their own source of pain. I have known Ann for twenty years and she has been doing persistent work on her own mental and emotional healing, clearing out blockages of fear, resentment, and pain. She is loving, creative, and insightful. I am in awe of her amazing psychic ability to perceive past life and ancestral experiences, which probably could not have occurred without her clearing out the barriers of torment from her childhood."

—Arleen Carr, M.Ed.

This book is dedicated to all who have been harmed by sexual abuse.
It holds a message to all who have lived with sexual abuse.
Remember to protect and treasure yourself.
Know that you are not alone.
Believe in the future.

Disclaimer:

This book contains the opinions and experience of the author. It is intended to provide support for those living with the anguish of sexual abuse. These words and suggestions may be helpful in opening more paths to healing. There are no simple techniques that will unlock and heal the fear, mental and emotional trauma. Instead, the author offers her own experiences in hopes of encouraging others on their journey. The advice and strategies contained in the book may not be suitable for every situation. The author disclaims any responsibility for any liability, loss, or risk, either personal or otherwise, that occurs as a consequence, directly or indirectly, of the use and applications of the contents of this book. If professional assistance is required, the services of a competent professional person should be sought.

Acknowledgements / I Am Grateful

This is a learner's journey. I thank so many friends who have helped me heal with the writing. Thanks to Sybil Watts, who guided me in the beginning with technical support and help in organizing my experiences. Marjorie Issacs, one of my oldest and dearest friends, read and reread into my heart and my manuscript to bring clarity to both with her professional experience and love. I respect your professionalism. Arleen Carr often knows my thoughts before I do and offered valuable insights with the writing and my personal quest to grow up. Anne Conkin supported my spirit and words and was there when I needed her wisdom. Her life experiences enriched me and this book. Justin Meridith supported me when I needed photos on a windy day and technical computer support when I was beyond being logical. Thanks to Ronna Gil for the photo of me. George Taylor created a powerful cover. His professional experience was invaluable in so many ways. He rescued photos of the paintings, answered too many questions—particularly when I did not have the experience to make technical or wise decisions. Kenny, my partner, has been a support when it was not easy to be supportive. Perhaps we will play checkers again without my runaway emotions. I am not often a good loser when losing happens in succession. I am blessed to have many friends and family who have been with me in creating this book. I am grateful to all of you.

This is a prayer to all who have been touched or frightened in innumerable ways by sexual abuse. Believing that this slim book might have value kept me going when I was tired with the process of getting it completed. Is it possible that words can leap from the page and from my heart to yours? May you and I connect in a moment of trust. Hopefully these imperfect words have permission to surround you and comfort you in those deep places where pain and fear live. Many others have traveled the path to wholeness. You are not alone. Yet, your journey is unique. Know in your heart that your success touches many lives.

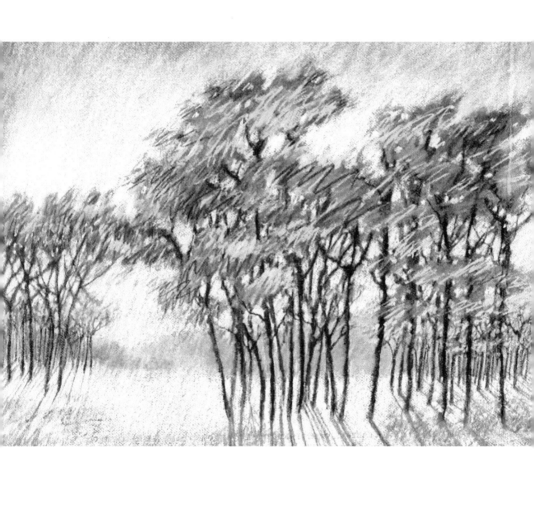

A Line of Trees Explored: Background of the Front Cover

This Line of Trees separates a troubled past from a brighter future. The opportunity to heal our lives is in the present, between the past and the future. All of us who have survived sexual abuse can move beyond the dark past that seems to push to the present of our consciousness. We can choose to live in the spacious, sunny, nourishing space of the present day. It is possible. There are openings we can walk through. The painful and difficult work of healing takes courage and support. This row of trees is like a barrier we can choose to overcome to reach an open space of light. There we can work on healing. This bright open space beyond where the trees part offers the choice to trudge through the shadows from the past and move beyond the pain. Clock and calendar time pass, yet we may still be living in the old shadows. Although the shadows may be scary, they are familiar, and one may simply survive day to day. This book offers an alternative, a path from the past into a brighter future. It has no miracle cure; instead it offers support on the journey. The shadows from the trees represent the present. This area of dark and light contrast offers an opportunity for making choices. Even the first step takes courage. Beyond the front row of trees is the future and unknown. There are additional rows of trees in the distance. They may indicate more opportunities for change and new learning. Growth is often a gradual happening; life continues to bring challenges that offer opportunities for change. Be brave and take the first step. Welcome nature; it is a healing power. Trees, plants, rocks, earth, animals, water, wind, sun, moon—all natural elements are gifts! They can bring comfort amidst the difficult work of healing.

An exploration into the significance of the photograph of Ann on the rocking horse is discussed later following the Introduction to Art Therapy and an Art Therapist's Journey.

An idea:

("An idea" will be offered at the end of each section with thoughts on how to support healing and suggest concrete creative ideas enlarging the concepts.) Sometimes it is difficult to acknowledge that there is a past, present, and future. The past is so powerful that it seems ready to explode into the present. The past shadows linger in the now. To think about a future can be very difficult because the video of the past keeps replaying over and over. To pause the video requires change and courage. To delete or repair the video requires a lot of work. Examining thoughts and memories is a decision to move beyond the past, reevaluate the present, and open to a new future. It is important to create a break or make a break from the shadows and the wall. It is impossible to delete the past. It may crowd into your mind yet it does not need to control your thoughts. You have power! Consider creating a mantra, a phrase that is an affirmation. An affirmation can be said over and over until the power comes into your heart. Begin simply. These are suggestions: "I will consider making a change in how I feel." "I am tired of being unhappy." "I am very afraid, yet I will think about a change I can try." "I have power." "I will protect myself." Then gradually build to "I love myself."

Later consider: "I have the power to seek wisdom and respect," or "I can protect myself and support others in their healing." Best of all is to create your own mantra! You might post it using a note on your bathroom mirror, refrigerator, computer, dashboard of your car. These words may not feel possible in the beginning. Instead, know that it has worked for others and can work for you! **BELIEVE.**

Note to Reader

Sexual abuse is not easy to write or talk about. Writing this book has taken me back in time, touching again my own pain. Too many lives have been tragically changed by sexual abuse. Abuse leaves people feeling isolated, very lonely, like "damaged goods," physically, mentally, emotionally, and spiritually wounded. It has been a problem since the beginning of time. Abuse touches women and men, girls and boys. It is an ancient story, yet it continues, until we decide "no more!"

The hopeful news is that since more people have come forward to speak of it, abuse is becoming a little easier to talk about. In this book, I share my own experience growing up not knowing about my abuse yet being aware of dysfunction in my life. I began this project of sharing because no one else can express my truth.

The pastels were painted as part of my own adult healing from sexual abuse twenty years ago. The paintings may be helpful to others who are healing from sexual abuse. Making art has advantages. Art work is safely contained by the edges of the paper while colors can bring intense emotions into focus. The feelings can also remain on the paper, protecting the self.

Expressing emotions through making art can make feelings easier to understand. Creating art helps quicken acceptance of the abuse, of the victim's innocence, and the understanding that recovery is possible. Finally, there is a separation from the emotions. The feelings are outside of the person's body, mind, and spirit and instead on paper or in another creative activity like clay, wood or words on paper. The paintings included in this book were made while I was working with a therapist during a difficult time, both emotionally and physically. After my therapy they were zipped into a black binder and forgotten until now. Know that some of these paintings are emotionally strong/intense. You have the option to skip some of them and come back to them later if you choose. You might have confusing/mixed emotions. It can be difficult. Healing is unique for each person. The process is gradual because there are so many levels of healing. It is not possible to simply speed through to recovery. Take time to think about who will support you and what activities may comfort you on this healing journey. Do you have a friend you can talk with about this work or anything else life throws at you? Some people can comfort, others may be too frightened to be involved with your journey but will support you in other ways like joining you at the grocery store. It is very important to have time boundaries around this work. It may be helpful to spend an hour working and then go for a walk with a friend or a friendly dog. Physical activity, like cleaning or exercise, yard work and gardening or sports, helps decrease anxiety. Find what works for you and it will help bring you back to daily life. Vigorous activity helps release anger. You might consider washing the kitchen floor or the bathroom. A warning! It is easy to be drawn to comfort foods, but over time healthy meals and snacks will help you feel better. Candy, cookies, fast foods, smoking, drugs, or alcohol will at first make you feel better, yet later will make you feel worse. If you are high on drugs, alcohol, or any addiction, you cannot connect to the feelings and concentrate on healing. Natural, healthy foods support your body, mind and spirit.

My journey has an outside story, which the therapist in me will tell, and an inside story which the "child within the paintings" will share. The process of healing is different for each person. I hope that my sharing will give courage to others on their journey. There is so much pain and confusion with sexual abuse. There is no simple answer or cure. Most important is to love yourself and feel whole, no matter what happened or how long ago it happened. Trusting and loving yourself opens you to healing and sharing love and trust with others. Healing may take a long time; it takes courage to go back, to uncover and work with those old wounds.

There are books on art therapy and abuse, many excellent books on the subject of sexual abuse.

This book begins with an introduction to art therapy. The healing that comes from creating art is pivotal to my story, to my life. The following is a rambling story of how the idea for this book evolved. The black-and-white photo of me on my rocking horse propelled the story into action, and the remainder is centered around the pastel paintings I did twenty years ago. Beginning paintings briefly describe some difficult aspects of growing up in our confusing, chaotic culture. The remainder of the paintings came from my work with a therapist, as I was clarifying what I had said or needed to say by letting the shapes and colors seep through me and at times explode onto the paper. Some days, I could not find or utter the words, yet what was essential came as images. Shapes and colors told my story then. Only now I can add words.

Growing up and healing can be scary at times. Be fearless. I promise you, your journey to wholeness will be worth it. You are special and important. Those who are wounded yet on a healing path can often help and encourage others in pain, especially those who are just beginning their work to wholeness.

"I send love to you." – Ann Owen

An idea:

Find something that brings you comfort. Sometimes, a special stone or another object that is small and fits in your hand can be a comfort. It might be special jewelry, a ring, belt, stone, scarf, or a piece of smooth or fuzzy fabric. The power of an object is immense. It is not the value but the emotional feelings connected to it that bring the magic. Think of clothes that have power. What color or texture might make you feel brave. What might you wear to protect yourself or help you "stand tall." Perhaps there might be a time when you need to hide—find clothes for blending in. Naturally it is not only the color but also the style, and that is a personal choice! This might become a treasure hunt. Resale shops are a wonderful place for experimenting and exploring a new you. Or, you might need those boots that are made for walking!

Table of Contents

The Importance of Art Therapy

As an art therapist, I often look at my world through the lens of my own artwork and creative expression around me. Art therapy is a way of communicating, recognizing, and using images and symbols. Engaging through art allows people to move beyond words, reasoned thoughts, and intellectual analysis to the underlying feelings. Unlike everyday conversation, communication in the therapeutic setting deals more directly with emotions. Feelings are honored by going beyond the verbal and intellectual understanding of life situations into the powerful emotions surrounding them. Art therapy helps one deal even more directly with anxiety, hurt, anger, fear, hatred, trauma and abuse, loss of brain function, or even loss of awareness and physical abilities caused by trauma and abuse. These emotionally charged areas are often forbidden in "polite society" or even the family. These very personal truths of the heart are scary. Resolving the problems they cause may take professional support.

I will paraphrase information from the American Art Therapy Association's handbook: *An art therapist has knowledge of human development, psychological theories, and training in visual arts and the creative process, which provides an inclusive approach for working with clients both young and adult.*

Art is important in my life. My parents met at the Art Institute of Chicago. Art was my favorite subject in school and I taught art in grade schools and on the college level. I became an art therapist. When I worked at Hospice, I often used art with clients, helping children and adults grieving the death of a loved one or facing their own death. When I worked in jail and prison with individuals and groups, art was included. The guards were always a little anxious when I entered those locked doors because I didn't sit quietly talking. Instead, I helped the prisoners act out solutions or make/create art to help them understand what caused some of their problems. This type of expression helped.

There are many techniques for understanding problems. There is never a "one size fits all" in art therapy or any counseling.

An idea:

Think about what is fun and creative for you. Is it sports, exercise, sewing, cooking, gardening, woodwork, writing, planning a holiday, adding color to an adult design or coloring book using colored pencils or pens? Give yourself time to explore the activity and keep the activity simple. Practice until you see what is fun and creative for you. Congratulate yourself and be proud of each of your successes. Is there someone you can share it with? Put a ribbon for your accomplishments and the flat art or photos of the creation, if possible, on your refrigerator. It might be a small step, yet small steps are important. Change happens with lots of small steps.

Introduction:
An Art Therapist's Journey

Recognizing Childhood Sexual Abuse /
Working on Healing:

This book has pastel paintings that may help children, parents, and therapists discover thoughts and feelings like the following:

- "Yes, I have known these feelings. It is scary to accept and talk about sexual abuse."

- "I have seen an image like that in dreams or maybe daydreams or nightmares, and I could not understand where it came from or why that image would be in my thoughts?"

- "I feel dirty!"

- "I wonder if I could somehow be guilty?"

- "How could something so terrible have happened to me when I cannot remember it?"

- "I remember too much, and I can hardly keep going, living a life that feels lonely and cruelly isolated."

- "I am so angry! I want to hurt certain people!"

- "I was so little and you didn't protect me."

All of these reactions and many others are accepted and respected. They are normal responses to non-normal events. Yet through therapy and your own ways of telling your story it is possible to heal and feel whole, clean, and free. An important step is to recognize the memories and express the truth in this pain. Verbalizing these feelings can help with letting go. Someday, it may even be possible to forgive the perpetrators, although forgiveness is not necessary to healing. This work is not easy, so it is OK to take your time. It is always possible to return to this work later, to see it with new eyes as you heal and encounter new life experiences. The healing work may need to be done over and over. Each day we may have new levels of awareness and understanding. With healing we can grow stronger and more self-loving. This is a process of going through time and space in your personal story. Working through these parts of my past, I realize that there was a purpose, a learning that was essential for my growth. I needed time to accept what had happened. Art therapy is part of my chosen way of learning. When you think about exploring such difficult memories, you may wonder, "Is the truth worth the pain?" It was for me.

The process of healing will be different for each person. These pastel paintings may be helpful to other survivors of sexual abuse, because color magnifies the intensity of the feelings, and my images may help to affirm your own. I believe and hope my paintings can help quicken emotional awareness and acceptance essential to recovery.

When I created the pastels, I was an adult and a professional artist, teacher, and therapist looking back at my own life. They were created when I felt pushed into therapy again because of physical problems with my eyes. The eyes are symbolic.

In therapy again, dealing with the sexual abuse, I made art to accompany my talking therapy. I worked with pastels because they are fluid and flexible. The benefit of using pastels is that I did not have to choose a particular brush depending on the space in the composition, mix paint, judge how much would be needed for a particular area, then let it dry before continuing to the next area. You get the idea: pastels are more immediate and spontaneous.

Now as I write, I realize that some of the images in the pastels seem to have pushed in from outside and beyond my awareness. When I found the courage to permit them to come through me, images exploded onto the paper. It was as if some belonged to other people and I was available to give them breath and life. I did not censor them, rather I worked to get them beyond me and onto paper. As I worked, I felt a unity with other survivors and their varied experiences, although this I did not understand at the time. I will share my insight about this concept later.

Looking back, I realize there were many techniques that helped my healing in addition to making art. Some of the things I did on the healing path included: talking with psychologists, therapists, family and friends; keeping dream journals; writing in diaries; being a member of various support groups like Al-Anon and a sexual support group; and now writing this book.

It seems impossible that I didn't realize I had been sexually abused. However, I was very young when it happened. Finally, talking with my sister jolted me into realizing and acknowledging the unaccepted and unacceptable truth. I had been sexually abused by my father.

All the years before acknowledging the abuse, I was healing different aspects and problems of living. They were important and the time was not wasted. I share my story because in the process of remembering and healing, more acceptance, love, trust, and joy became available to me. Looking again at the paintings, the images, colors, textures, shapes, and relationships of objects helped bring memories and feelings to the surface and the light of day, where they could be reexamined. Self-protection can keep memories, too scary to even think about, lost and hidden in the unconscious. These old, hidden memories can influence current life without a person understanding what is happening. What is hidden or unacknowledged can be very destructive. That is what happened to me. Those unhealed memories in my unconscious continued to create problems in my life, my health, my happiness. It was difficult to trust people or situations. "I" developed a problem with my "eye," which was my final push into therapy, creating the paintings and seeing the truth. During my career, I often pushed through challenges. One of my professors in the Master's of Visual Arts program asked me why I wanted the degree since I would never be hired on the college level. Women didn't get those jobs. I was both really sad and really mad. The mad won! I was hired several years later with the help of friends. One example of how I held myself back was three years before I retired, I had the opportunity to apply for "Full Professor" yet was afraid to try. It took a lot of pushing from my husband to begin the process. The approval process is very competitive. Full of self-doubt, I analyzed years of teaching to prove my worth. I had exhibited in many art shows and won awards. The most was $1,000. Yet, I wasn't sure how an exhibit of Spirit Boxes I made, which were inspired by a trip to Thailand, would compare to professors who published books. Friends of mine had tried for "Full Professor" but were denied although they had accomplished impressive work. Somehow, I had to prove first to myself and then to the Humanities Division faculty that I was worthy. Only a few applications move on to higher levels of evaluation. To my surprise, my document went through the Humanities Division, the entire college, and on to the university for recognition. I was honored to become a Full Professor. I laid open my heart and was rewarded.

After working on sexual abuse with a therapist and feeling better, I zipped the paintings into a black portfolio. They eventually got lost in my collections of drawings and paintings. I no longer wanted to be reminded of the grief. I moved that black portfolio, with the images carefully hidden and zipped inside, from one home to another, four times through the years. They were part of the baggage I carried with me. The paintings were forgotten and ignored as I tried to deny and hide the story—the truth of my past.

There were still dysfunctional parts of my life, although I was much freer and happier than before therapy. Finally, during the latest move, which included downsizing at age eighty-three, I realized that I needed to make a decision: either burn the paintings or print them in a book. No one would want to hang them on a wall or in an exhibition, yet burning does not delete the experience. It remains seared in the memory. The latter decision meant writing my story. Which also meant, once again, bringing those painful memories to the surface, to continue healing. Healing is a multilayered process. Life keeps happening between the times of healing, and I required more adjustments with new understanding. I needed to go back in time to understand some of my early signs of dysfunction before I discovered and admitted my sexual abuse.

I am going to digress and tell a little of my background that helps to explain some of my dysfunction. Growing up I sometimes felt little, lonely, confused, and sometimes ugly. I did not really feel alive in my body except when I danced. I did not trust my body, myself and especially any males. I did not feel close to my father, although I didn't know why. That was simply my reality. I tried hard to be a good daughter, studying hard and getting mostly A's and B's. However, school seemed much easier for my sisters. This was when I began comparing myself to others. I was the oldest, yet I compared myself to my younger sisters and sometimes I fell short. Actually, in real life, I was secretary of my high school senior class of over four hundred students; yet, I did not consider myself popular. Often I did not like myself, especially when comparing myself with others. I was uncomfortable. It was an inner game of *"was I good enough?"* or sometimes *"better than others?"* even though others didn't know the game.

When nineteen, I got married to leave home and quickly became pregnant. When my second child was still a baby we moved across the country to California, leaving behind the support of my friends and family. Soon I had three beautiful children, each separated by two years. As a wife and mother, I was immature and confused. Yet, somehow, I stumbled through being a mother and struggling to become an adult. It took a lot of practice and learning. It was a lonely time. As soon as my youngest was in school, I completed a teaching credential and began teaching kindergarten. I felt comfortable working with young children who would not challenge me.

There were good times and bad times as my children and I grew up. During this period I completed a master's degree in art in Mexico. I suspected divorce was coming long before it happened. Yet, it was a shock because suddenly, I had to be completely responsible for myself and my middle child. My oldest was enrolled in a university far away, and my youngest joined his father. I was losing a husband and my best friend, who was his new wife, my youngest son, plus all of my support system. I moved into a new beginning.

Although life was difficult after the divorce, I became a quick learner and was blessed with great opportunities. I was accepted into the Expressive Art Therapy Master's program and I was offered a teaching position at the community college. Both were the perfect challenge and opportunity. I had read about art therapy years before, and at that time it became a dream for the future. The program was both a learning experience and personal therapy when I really needed it!

One of the standard things an art therapist student learned was how to administer and analyze the House, Tree, Person Projective Drawings. The concept behind it was that all three drawings were symbols for the individual. When people make these pictures, they project their conscious and even unconscious feelings into the drawings. When I did the House, Tree, Person Drawings myself, I could see problems. The tree had few limbs on the left, which symbolized the past. I linked those signs in my drawings to my recent divorce. The front of the house was very simple, which at the time was the honest truth. I was renting a small place with a concrete floor and little amenities. The person looked very tired and fearful. That, too, was my reality. I was surviving on four hours of sleep with teaching and going to classes. I could justify everything!

Being at peace with my divorce offered me the opportunity to focus on my career. In the beginning I had a lot of pain and anger to work through. My first husband and I are friends today. We talk on the phone and worry about our grown children and grandchildren. I learned a lot in my first marriage.

Too soon, I jumped into a second marriage. Quickly, I realized that I had married an alcoholic. Naively, I thought love could change him. Soon my magical thinking was gone. AA and Al-Anon saved me; saved us both. A wonderful therapist, who at the time made me very angry, warned me I could not leave this marriage until I'd completed two years in Al-Anon! Otherwise, he promised, I would repeat the same situation and experience the same problems again. I trusted his word and became dedicated to attending Al-Anon twice a week. I learned more about being responsible for myself, acknowledging my boundaries and protecting myself. Equally important, I learned I could permit myself and others to fail. Even though, in the beginning, I did not want to attend those meetings, after almost eighteen years in Al-Anon, I had to admit it was truly a blessing. Friends in Al-Anon became family. Through the AA programs my husband and I discovered we did not want to be divorced. Together, he and I became more independent and loving and were happily married for nineteen years. With support, he conquered alcoholism, smoking, and diabetes and died later on his own terms. He chose not to have chemo or radiation and instead was surrendered by the love of family and grandchildren.

During my late fifties, I had a problem with my right eye rolling up into my skull. For a while I had double vision. Later, I could only see with my left eye. I wore a black patch, stumbled a lot, and had trouble driving the forty-five minutes back and forth to work and home. I was very tired all the time. Of course, the right eye got worse. During that time I began losing teeth and my body seemed to be falling apart. I paid a friend to grade papers at the college where I taught art. Finally, since doctors were not able to find a diagnosis for what was happening, the school offered me early retirement—perhaps because I had never taken a sabbatical where they paid for time away from teaching. With my husband's support I had the time and motivation—no, it was desperation—to begin therapy again, looking deeper into the secrets of my childhood. My eye problems became a metaphor for understanding my early childhood with more clarity. I had to see what my heart knew, yet my eyes were previously not able, or not willing, to see. This was a time of tears, writing, working with dreams, making the pastel paintings in this book, and talking with another excellent therapist. I began healing: mind, body, emotions, and spirit, which continues to this day.

The time was right because my three children were grown and successful in their own careers. I began to realize that I had been affected for most of my life by what had happened when I was a baby. Suddenly, without my career, there was time and motivation to return to the source, through the tears and fears. The paintings would sometimes scare me; yet, I continued making art. Images flowed in and I did not censor them. They were both mine and seemed to be more than my remembrances. They might have come from sisters and brothers, now or in the past, or someone next door. I opened my heart, cried over the images and memories, and gave voice to them in color, shape, texture, and in relationship to each other. I did not understand all the symbols; their meanings are magical and they grow, change, and continue to develop. Voices from the images came later to help me decipher the symbolism. Today, I understand more deeply. I still feel twinges of fear and anxiety seeing the paintings; yet, I am not overwhelmed, encased, or smothered by them. The paintings help me now by showing me how far I have come.

I accept that I can't "delete" the past! Unfortunately, in the last move of downsizing, I burned diaries and journals, tapes, and even the black robe I wore as a professor going down the aisle in many graduations. I was clearing out the past, ready to be lighter and begin anew again. I did not destroy the black portfolio. The paintings were an important part of my therapy, and the portfolio moved along with my other collections of baggage. Even now, many years later, the power of the images comes through and brings tears as I recall difficult times. Looking at them these days, sometimes my stomach gets tight and I need to break away from the intensity. Other times, these paintings seem like children calling out for help. I send love to them, to myself, to "the little girl within," and all who are still suffering and have suffered. These paintings have helped me move through the old fears.

Know that the recovery process can help you, whatever techniques you choose, to open yourself to support and love.

As a therapist, I often help others support their "child within." I will explain this process because it can be very powerful. Sometimes when we are hurt, we wall off the pain by trying to forget. We may lose awareness of the trauma, but its symptoms continue to haunt us. If, instead of misplacing awareness, we decide to face the painful truth and make necessary changes, then life can become simpler and more peaceful. I often use hypnosis. I completed the hypnosis credential because it worked well with the intuitive aspects of art therapy. You can do some work on your own. Promise yourself to contact a therapist if things seem overwhelming or frightening.

The following is a simplified approach to helping the "child within." First, spend time relaxing. Trust that whatever comes to you has value even when it is difficult to understand. Intention is the most important asset, although prayer and meditation may help. If you had a childhood name or nickname, use it. That childhood name is very powerful for going back in time. You can have a conversation with your younger self. In therapy it becomes a three-way conversation: client, child, and therapist. As you do this work, keep thinking, "Yes, I can trust whatever happens." Experiment. Practice. If you get stuck, ask:

"When did things change? When did life become so difficult: college or university or on a job? High school? Middle school? Grade school? Toddler? Baby?" The answer may come intuitively or you might use a pendulum. Getting this information is enough for a beginning. When talking with your "child within" using the old nickname, the child-hood name, ask if your child is willing to continue exploring the past. Promise to support and love them, whatever comes, whether it seems to make sense or not. You may imagine hugging or holding your young self, the "child within." Ask both your younger self and your today self, "Are you willing to trust this process?"

Sometimes, the child has been so frightened and wounded that it takes time to build trust. If so, then first, take more time to learn what your child liked to do. Who could they trust? Where did they go or hide when afraid? What made them happy? Finally, just talk or write. You might describe more about yourself so your child will understand the situation in the present. This helps bridge past and present, which is very important. After sharing, ask if your little one wants more visits. Most importantly, ask if your child is willing to promise to share when they are afraid. Your child might get frightened when your present life gets tough. With fear, anger, or confusion in your present life, your "child within" might be anxious. Take time to check in. How can the "child within" let you know when they need support? The trigger or call for help may be a tightness in your stomach, an intuitive feeling, or even fear. It might happen when you suddenly see a color that is symbolic like red for anger, hear a song that your body reacts to from the past, recognize an image that reclaims power, enjoy a memorable taste, identify a smell with a history, remember sensing a texture or touch. For example, apple pie or chocolate ice-cream cones might hold wonderful associations or have painful memories attached. The treat may have a mixed message. When confusion happens, it is wise to promise to check inside, trust your intuition, and take time to comfort the "child within." Ask the child what they want to do: walk in the park, sing songs, take a bubble bath, read a book, talk with a friend, make a craft project, play softball, color with crayons, or whatever safe activity comforts the "child within." Promise support and protection because this "child within" is so precious and important, both then and now. Honor your feelings.

These are suggestions that have worked for me. They require patience and practice. The key ingredients are trust, support, and the intention to grow.

An idea:

*Work with a notebook or journal. 1. **Write** memories or stories or dreams that are important. This is not for showing to anyone. It is your private journey that you can hide unless or until it feels good to share it. Write as much as you can remember. It is helpful to get the words outside of yourself, no matter how angry or ugly or painful. There is no judgement. It helps to have paper, pen, and a flashlight beside your bed. Writing helps you remember dreams. 2. **Find photos**, magazine images, or pictures on the Web that remind you of an event. Collect them in the journal and if they are disturbing, scribble all over them to hide the image or fold them over until you are ready to look at them. You are the one in control of when and even if you choose to face those things. Next, to give yourself some additional power over the memories/images, decide if it is helpful to keep them. 3. **Create a ceremony** that traces your journey starting at an important time and continuing as you grow stronger. 4. **Dance and move**. Find hip-hop, jazz, symphonic or folk music that helps tell your story. 5. **Decorate a box or envelope**. You can make it very, very ugly or powerful, protective or beautiful to hide what is inside. Then put anything related to the abuse in it. It is your decision if you choose to keep it, hide, bury, or burn it.*

These ideas can help the process of recovery step by step. The journey is not quick or easy. It takes courage. Since you are already reading this book, you already are showing more courage than you might have thought possible.

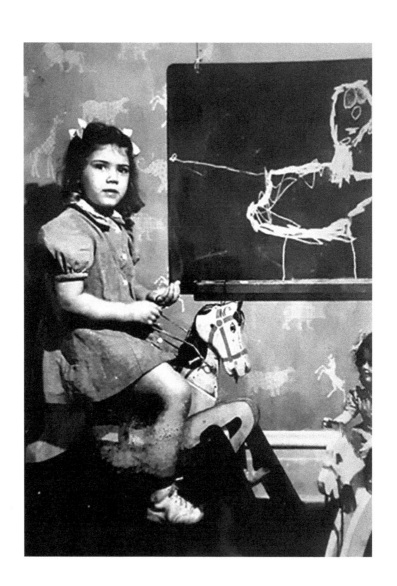

Ann on Her Rocking Horse with Drawing

Recently, this little black-and-white photo of me fell out of an envelope with a letter, from at least 25 years ago, that had never been mailed. I had the equipment and opportunity at the college to copy old family photos and surprise family with our past history. What a miracle to find it now!

I was formally posed on my rocking horse and in the lower right corner, my favorite doll, Deana Durban, on a smaller horse. Above her on the chalkboard is my drawing. This is the most important part of the photograph. The drawing has signs of unknown problems in the way a young child can speak without words simply using lines and shapes. The art therapist in me sees that I was trying to protect my body in the drawing with the many surrounding "protecting" lines. The eyes are very large but look almost blank or surprised and shocked. The face expresses fear and confusion? The throat is blocked with lines, disconnecting the head and body so the head cannot know what is happening to the body? Plus, being disconnected, the head cannot talk with the body, cannot understand what risk/dangers the body senses. The tiny right hand is much smaller than the eyes and has no fingers to help protect the body. It looks helpless, yet reaches to the edge of the blackboard. Is it reaching for help? The arm is a single, ragged, elongated, scraggly line. The same single lines suggest legs with no feet to hold up a very heavy body. The art therapist in me can see the signs of abuse in that chalk drawing made almost eighty years ago. Analyzing the photo helped me accept in my heart that I had been abused. How scared and sad I feel looking at the photo. "I can protect you now, little one!"

How old was I then? Maybe five years old? What was happening at that time? I can only guess. "I love you very much. You are precious! Now I am with you and you are with me!"

Like many survivors of abuse, owning my truth has happened on different levels over time. With each new acceptance, I feel more empowered and trusting of myself. This book can help support survivors on their journey. The book offers survivors, parents, and therapists visuals that speak powerfully and offer material for discussion.

An idea:

Add in a notebook, along with any memories from the abuse, words that you were never allowed to say like: "I hate you!" "You are so ugly, everything about you is ugly!" "I will never trust or believe anything you say again!" "I wish you would die!" You might find a pillow or get one at a secondhand store that you can pound. Take it to a safe place and pound and pound it. You can also try using a baseball bat to pound the pillow. The physical attack on a pillow can be empowering for releasing emotions.

Pastel Paintings

These paintings were made over fifty years ago when I was working with a therapist and finally dealing with my sexual abuse. This section contains pastel paintings that symbolize various types of abuse: verbal, physical, emotional, mental, spiritual, and sexual. Some are scary.

I encourage you to continue your journey of recovery. The work will be difficult, yet only you can do it to make a difference in your life. It takes courage, a special strength you do have, even if you don't recognize or feel it right now. After all, you did survive all the trouble. Put on your tall boots and begin.

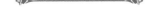

Part I. Difficult Family Relationships

The first three paintings focus on family interaction. Take time to look at the first three paintings. It might be helpful to write down some of your feelings. Then choose the questions you want to think about today from the list below. You can choose some of these questions each time you look at paintings in this book.

- What are the different people doing?
- How are they reacting to each other?
- Can you guess what each one is feeling?
- What might they be saying?
- How do you feel about the situation?
- Have things like this happened to you?
- What would you say if you were in this situation?
- Would you be brave enough to say how you feel?
- How was your family different?

If you write about feelings now, it may surprise you to see if later your feelings change. Each one of us sees different things and reacts differently to the situations because of our backgrounds. There is no right or wrong answer. I was surprised to learn that some friends felt differently than I do about my paintings. How each one of us reacts depends on what we have experienced, and even that can change over time. How we react when we are young is different than when we grow older. Another change can happen when we have more power to protect ourselves or experiences that help us deal with emotional relationships. By taking one step, we gain strength to take another.

The first three paintings focus on dysfunctional family relationships.

An idea:

Choose one of the family situations that might have been true for you and your family. Use your notebook or a sheet of paper. Draw a table—square or circle—and draw an X or O for each person in your family and add their names. Or, draw your family doing something. Or find photos in a magazine that might symbolize your family and paste them on a paper doing something. Write about what might have happened and how you felt, who you were next to, who you felt safe with, and who you could not trust. Scribble over the drawing if you get angry. If your situation is different, both describe it and how you felt. Write what you wish you could have said. How would that have made a difference? Can you guess how other people might have reacted?

Maybe try drawing a map of where the abuse happened. See what memories come. If it is too scary, stop and tear up the paper and throw it away or burn it. Later you can try again; being concrete might help make the details clearer.

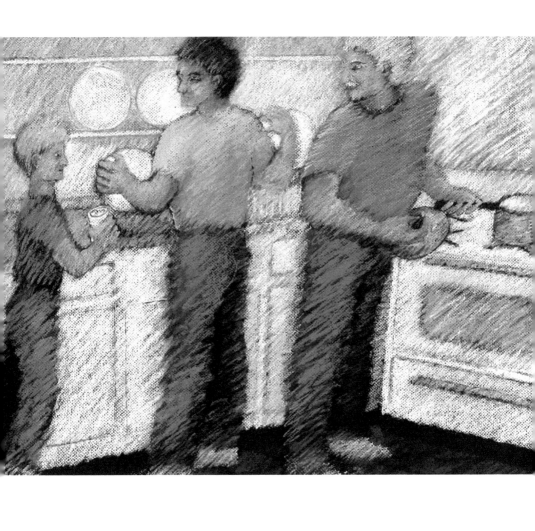

Boy Asking for Milk/Seeking Love

The following three paintings focus on family interaction. Take time to look at them. I will repeat some of the questions listed earlier.

- What do you see?
- What are the different people doing?
- How are they reacting to each other?
- What might each person say?
- Can you guess what each person is feeling?
- Who is standing next to each other?
- What can you guess about their personalities?
- How do you feel about the situations?
- Have you known situations like this?

Choose what seems important to you.

It might be helpful to write some of your feelings in a journal. Have things like this happened to you? If your life was different, what happened? If you write about feelings now, it may surprise you later to see if your feelings have changed.

The young boy looks small, asking for attention. It feels as if his presence creates conflict. His request for milk expresses his hope for comfort and love.

The parents are like a wall of opposition to the young boy. There is a lot of tension and little compassion in the kitchen. The boy does not have the power to protect himself or to make changes in his relationship with the adults. All he can do is disappear, maybe hide, be angry, plan revenge.

Verbal abuse can be overwhelming. It makes you feel little, even stupid, ugly, and helpless. This dynamic may get worse without help from outside. This is especially true if there is no support from the larger family of aunts, uncles, and grandparents who do not live nearby.

Sometimes school, church, or groups like Boy and Girl Scout clubs, the YMCA, or good neighbors or friends can make a difference in supporting children.

An idea:

In your notebook, consider writing about the abuse you felt growing up. It might be that older siblings teased you and made you cry? Do you live with your parents now or did you at that time? Do you have other family members in your home? Has someone hurt your feelings or bullied you or beat you up? Is there someone you can talk with? Sometimes it is difficult for parents or other people to believe you when you try to talk about a problem, especially abuse. The situation may be complex and they might be afraid for themselves when trying to change things. Do you have grandparents who can help? Who else might help?

Were you the first child in the family? Second? Each child in the family has different responsibilities, problems, and even personality traits. The oldest needs to grow up, be responsible, and help babysit. The middle is sometimes lost in between and needs to grow up fast to make way for the next baby. The youngest can be a baby and everyone takes care of them. How was your relationship different with each person? Think about how this influences you even now. You might write your thoughts about what would make your life better. If you don't feel comfortable doing this now, come back to this idea later. It would be helpful to draw stick figures or cut out images from a magazine to tell your story. Using images sometimes lets you see more information or understand in a new way. With cut out shapes you can move them around until the relationships feel correct for your situation.

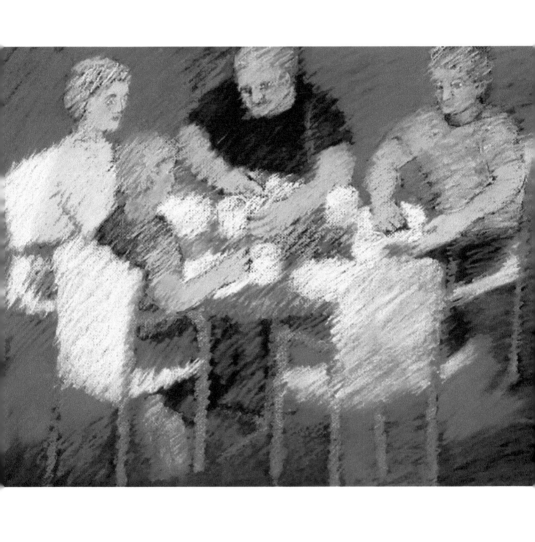

Family Dinner

The family is eating together, which hopefully is positive. Often people grab food and disappear into their own spaces, or watch TV or get immersed on their phones or games. Many people go out to eat, often for fast food instead of healthy vegetables, fruits, and proteins.

It feels like there is a lot of tension around the table. The boy might feel lonely, isolated, picked on. It is difficult, probably impossible for the boy to trust these adults. Sometimes this type of situation includes physical repercussions. He might wonder what is wrong with himself, what did he do that was so bad? Later, he could plot how to win his parents' respect and understanding, or plot to get even for his pain and fear.

Some of our young people and some adults make plans to end their life when tensions become overwhelming. Although these plans might feel like the only solution at the moment, hopelessness is a feeling, not a fact. There are ways to discover meaningful alternatives. Suicidal thoughts and gestures must be taken seriously. Normal growing up tension is complex enough. The typical questions may include: Who am I? How am I similar to my parents? How am I different? Why do I feel I do not belong? Was I adopted?

Confusion and fear can be multiplied by social media and its constant pressure. Bullying can be devastating. Belonging to a peer group becomes so important as children are growing up. The peer group can be a positive or negative influence. The Web presents opportunities and dangers. Parents need to be available to support and supervise young people, even as they strive to become independent. Growing up takes time, patience, and love, along with structure and support.

An idea:

What was mealtime like in your home? Did everyone help? Did peo-ple eat at the table? Was the TV going? Did you always sit in the same place? Did everyone have chores at home? What happened outside your home to influence how you feel today? Write or be creative, dance, draw, or make music, or find a video or a game that tells your story. You might create a comic character or an animal for each per-son. Who is like an elephant, a mouse, a fearless princess, or an evil ninja? There are games on the Web that let you act in powerful sce-narios. They might permit you to explore options. The danger is that many people, especially children. become addicted to the games and they escape into a fantasy world. Growing up is difficult.

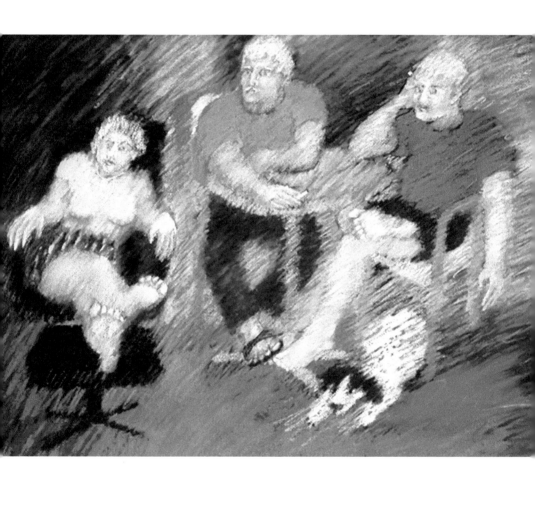

Family Relaxing

The family is intently watching TV, although the boy is absent. In the previous paintings, the boy was isolated; now he is not even present. Everyone stares vacantly in the glare of the TV. Today, some people get lost in their big-screen TV, their games, phone, or computer. Hours are lost on social media, video games, or shut off from conversation by earbuds while listening to their private music. Only the dog seems alert.

Many low-income families live in very crowded spaces, with little or no privacy. They are glad to have a roof over their heads. Often there is a constant bombardment of sound, comings and goings of people, sometimes strangers. Nothing is private. There is barely space to breathe. Sometimes there is not even space for your own bed or a spot to keep treasures safe. Higher-income families face a different situation where each child often has their own bedroom isolated from parents and siblings. Space can be good; space can also be lonely within four walls.

Some young people turn to drugs to numb themselves. Getting high protects them from feeling the pain of isolation and possible abuse, while allowing them, for a short time, to escape from reality. However, the danger is that they easily become addicted. Too often they may scheme to leave home as soon as possible. The way that seems easiest might be the most dangerous.

Life today is very complex. Growing up is not easy. It is difficult to find heroes beyond comic books, computers and videos. Many people bottle up their fear, pain and anger. With all the suppressed emotions, violence can erupt easily especially with so much violence on TV, in our neighborhoods, cities, nation, world. Yet, hope is available. Try counseling, education, reading widely to gain new information.

Creative activities like writing, dancing, playing sports, making art and music give people a way to express themselves and inspire others. In some of these activities the team can support each individual. Simple activities like being in nature can be rewarding. Enjoying plants, trees, the sunrise and sunset give an added level of meaning to each day. Friendship, prayer, religion, and meditation can support growth, a sense of belonging, and a feeling of peace. Sometimes the easiest thing is to sit, close your eyes, slow your breath, and be aware of each breath in and out. Include soft music. Imagine people or things you love. It might be a puppy or kitten you always wanted or a best friend.

An idea:

What helps you feel happy and at peace? What kind of music do you enjoy? Is there a special song that helps you feel happy? A quiet place in nature? Playing basketball, swimming laps, lifting weights, running, dancing, walking your dog, or loving your cat and listening to it purr—all these things can make a difference when life seems difficult. Prayer or meditation offers a quiet power. Doing something creative like making and decorating cupcakes and sharing them with someone, maybe the grouchy old lady next door or the lonely kid down the block, can bring joy to both you and them. When you reach out to other people, it may make a huge difference in their lives and in yours. You have the power to make a difference!

PART II. MY JOURNEY

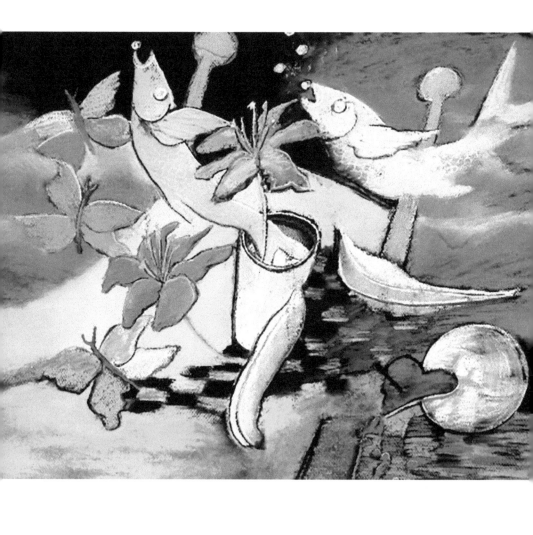

Milk and Bananas

This painting has a story that explains the abstract relationships. It goes back to a day in kindergarten. As a kid, I often enjoyed exploring and testing limits. Even now, I test limits in myself, as well as any limits that seem unfair. One day when I was in kindergarten, I went down a special slide in the schoolyard that was meant for older children. It was a slide with no sides or railings. You wrapped your legs around two sloping poles, and tried not to fall through the space between them. My mother warned me never to go on that slide. Naturally, I experimented on it and I fell. My wrist was broken and had to be in a cast. That was an unexpected expense for my family, already financially stretched during the days after the Depression. My parents were upset with me. I got spanked, and sent to bed with no dinner. Later, my father brought me a glass of milk and a banana. I refused both! Even today, I do not drink milk or eat bananas. Bananas are too similar to a penis.

In the right corner of the painting is a circle suggesting a crystal glass ball with my father's image coming in through the door. He feels menacing. Next to the glass ball is a heart, my heart, with a nail through it. My relationship with my father had always been distant. Before he died and before I acknowledged my sexual abuse, I could only imagine his back to me while he worked at his desk at home. I felt rejected and didn't know why I couldn't talk with him. Now, I guess that he was confused inside his heart. My best memories of my father were those times when he sang us to sleep. Years later, we sang those songs at his grave site.

Some more symbols in the painting are the poles. They may represent a goal post or bed post or relate to the slide in kindergarten. The checkerboard may be part of an unknown game of winners and losers? Checkers is still a difficult game for me today; I often lose because I can't plot future moves. Luckily, the fish are free and swimming away. The flowers are becoming butterflies and that is a positive sign, a symbol of transformation. Even then I was beginning to separate myself from painful feelings.

An idea:

What images stick in your mind? Maybe you try to forget them and they keep popping into your mind or into your dreams? They replay again and again. Sometimes, it helps to look in a magazine and find images that might help tell a little of your story. Cut them out and find more photos that fit together to tell your story. (The doctor's office may have old magazines you can use. Sometimes grocery stores have magazines they give away at the front door.) I glue the stories together on paper or poster board. These collage stories can be fun or scary. I have learned important information that I didn't realize consciously until I used this process. You don't need to show your artwork to anyone.

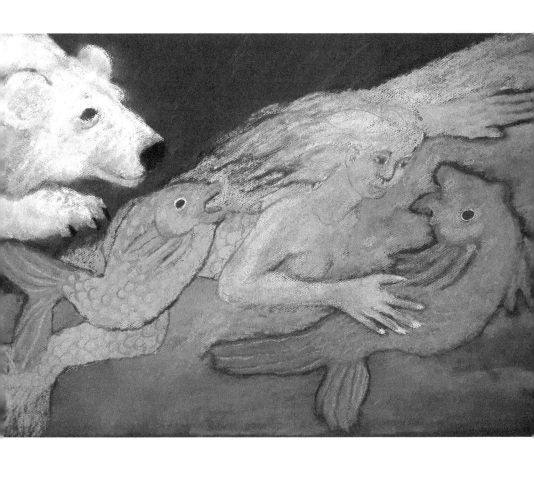

Mermaid Swimming with Fish

This pastel painting expresses freedom in the water. Carl Jung wrote that water is also a symbol of the unconscious. Events of our lifetime are stored in our unconscious, like a personal library. Some happenings are essential for who we are in our daily life, so we remember them. Other memories and feelings are hidden from our consciousness because they are not important, are too scary, upsetting, or do not fit with what we want others to believe about us. I lived most of my life not accepting the most scary ... sexual abuse.

As a child, I often trusted animals more than humans. Growing up, my family always had a dog and a cat. I have loved many dogs and cats. The animals I knew were trusting and loving. They always listened, never judged, and loved me unconditionally.

Over twenty years ago I became interested in power animals. I was attending drumming circles and sweat lodges that were patterned after Native American traditions. The ceremonies included many prayers for the earth, all the elements, animals, and people. Native peoples everywhere traditionally honor and respect the natural world and live in harmony with Mother Earth. They honor the stories and wisdom of the past. People work with power animals that are spirit guides. The spirits of the animals are an integral part of the people's daily lives. A person may have several power animals; I feel connected to polar bear, dolphin, and red-tailed hawk. When I need comfort and protection, I call on polar bear. When dealing with the unconscious or difficult situations, I call on the wisdom of dolphin. For an overall or higher vision or for travel, I call on hawk. To connect with my power animals, I close my eyes and imagine they are with me. I see them in my mind's eye, in my imagination, their fur or skin or wings; I sense that I can look into their eyes and feel their breath and heartbeat. They

MERMAID SWIMMING WITH FISH

protect me and I honor them. Even today I say a prayer when I see a dead animal and I always salute a hawk when I see one.

Animals keep sneaking into my paintings, including my personal power animals. On some occasions, I carefully plan a painting, working and reworking them. More often they develop spontaneously. Usually, I swim with dolphins when I visualize a healing journey that includes the unconscious. However in this painting the mermaid is swimming with salmon or goldfish. There is something sacred about the way salmon swim upstream to spawn new life. Perhaps the mermaid is looking for new hope and a new beginning? Polar bear is there to comfort. As I began my healing journey from sexual abuse, I needed my power animals.

An idea:

Choose a power animal. There is no right or wrong choice. Often your power animal is already an animal you feel close to. Every creature has powers that can be very useful. Ants work together cooperating on huge projects. Bees are amazing in how the community is essential and the queen bee is the center of the hive. There are books and Web programs that explain an animal's power. What powers does your animal possess? You probably know without any research. You may have more than one power animal, or they may work with you for a while and when your situation changes, a new animal may arrive. It is possible to work with a unicorn or a dragon or an animal you create. Imagine a conversation with your animal. If you are writing, use your dominant hand to write your questions and your nondominant hand for the animal's answers. It may sound kind of crazy! It is often a surprise what you learn. It takes trust to do something so strange as to imagine an animal talking, but you have probably felt a pet communicating feelings of love and protection. I no longer feel comfortable going to a zoo because I imagine the animals talking. I feel sorry they are in cages.

19

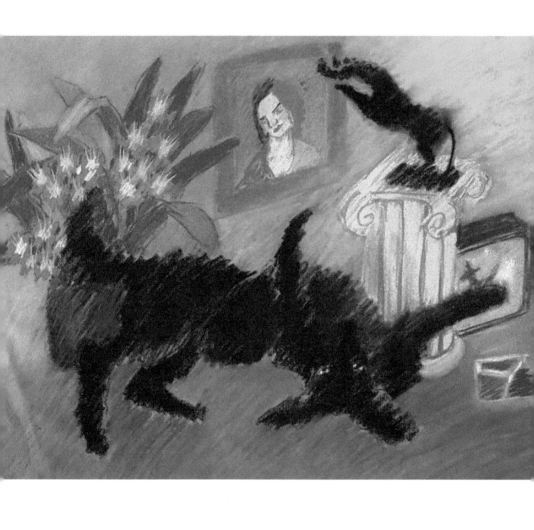

Black Dog Rolling on the Floor

The next two paintings of my big black dog are symbolic of my need for protection, support, and comfort. This loving, protective, big poodle died long ago.

In the first painting, my dog is rolling on the floor. He is being blessed by the sculpture of a hand above him. This black metal hand was cast from a Buddhist statue in India. The "Blessing Hand" is symbolic for me, and brings me joy. I am in the picture on the wall behind the hand, looking down at my big black poodle. There is another image of a dog on the TV, almost hidden by a paw. That dog is running free. I think that my poodle would love to run and play, but I need her for protection as I work in therapy on my abuse. There is an aluminum tray with dog food to keep her nourished and on the job. She loves and comforts me. I know that animals love people so much that sometimes they develop symptoms like their owners, to try to protect them.

Objects and words have power. When I feel vulnerable, I carry a crystal in my pocket and I have larger crystals around my home. I talk to plants inside my home and outside. Prayers are a traditional, powerful form of protection. Other forms of protection are affirmations and healing white light. These healing techniques were not taught in my home growing up; now they are part of my life of healing myself and others.

An idea:

What will bring you comfort, support, and protection? Create a safe place where you live. A personal safe place may be in a small corner or on a shelf. It might be in a box that you decorate and even hide if you want to. It may hold special rocks, stones, shells, dried flowers, photos of a place you want to visit or people you admire, or something you really want like a photo of a new car or words from an advertisement that will help you lose or gain weight. You can wear a special color when you need to be especially brave. A piece of jewelry or a ring or a stone, or a piece of furry fabric in your pocket can bring a calming presence. Affirmations protect, offer comfort, and are empowering. Some powerful affirmations are: "I am surrounded by love," "Angels guide me," "I make wise decisions." Make up your own and put it on your bathroom mirror, the refrigerator, the dashboard of your car. Say the affirmation when you stop for a red light or brush your teeth.

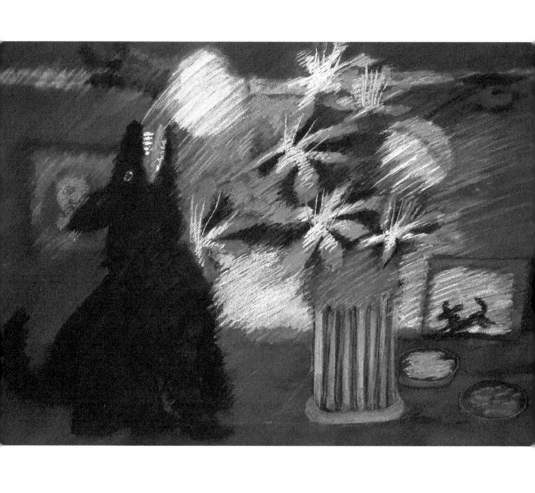

Howling Dog

I do not understand this painting. There are two yellow shapes that might be the sun and moon. Is my dog howling at the sun? The moon? Are they in the sky or are they in my living room? Is the light a symbol for new understanding or healing coming to me? The flowers are open, blooming. Why now? Maybe my dog is howling for me, expressing my anger, my helplessness, my lack of power. Perhaps, she is on duty at all times. I feel separated from her fierce emotions and powerful teeth. Her food and water are waiting until she can spare the time for herself. The dog on the TV is still running free and jumping off the screen. I am watching from the painting on the wall, not really involved in the confusion or even aware of the present happenings. Perhaps, I am not even present in my body?

Comments from Marjorie Isaacs, Psy.D.

Resolving trauma or abuse is difficult because it means facing confusing things. Our experiences were not what we expected. They were not normal. Reactions to these non-normal events can be hard to accept. Facing any part of the mixed-up world of abuse is a struggle. Separating in different ways is one way to get through it. Feeling distant from the facts or the feelings can keep people safer at the time. Whatever actually happened, you have a right to your own sense of it and any feelings you have about it.

Question for the Reader:

Maybe you have more ideas about what is happening in the painting? Everyone has their own interpretation of symbols because everyone's experiences are different. I thought I knew what the paintings meant because they came from my heart. I was surprised to learn that people saw different things and different meanings in these paintings. Maybe some of what is uncovered in these images can help you discover more understanding in your journey of recovery.

Do you feel emotions that seem disconnected from what you think or know happened? Sometimes, we reconstruct events to protect ourselves. Sometimes, we separate from ourselves or create a story that protects us and might not be as accurate. We might even float away to a safe place, away from what is happening to our body. We can protect ourselves in many ways. Healing requires being honest with both feelings and facts. Healing is not easy!

An idea:

*How do you express your feelings of helplessness? Do you get angry and lash out or scream, throw things, try to hurt other people? Do you hide, cry, become very defensive, blame others? Do you hurt yourself? Do you sometimes get so depressed that you want to die? Know that help is available. Suicide Prevention **1-800-273-8255** (TALK) is available twenty-four hours every day. Both English and Spanish-speaking counselors are available. The people who answer the phone are professional counselors. "It is free and confidential support for people in distress. By July 2022, the FCC has designated **988** as the new nationwide number for the National Suicide Prevention Lifeline." There is hope and there is light that is available for everyone. Reach out to trusted people. Who or what keeps shining in your life and helps you smile when you explore dark things like trauma or abuse?*

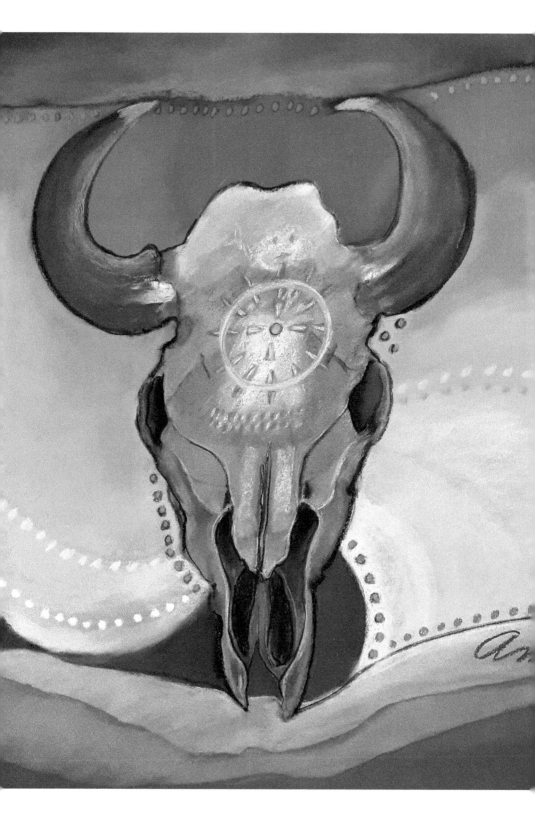

Buffalo Skull

The buffalo skull is symbolic in Native American cultures. It is powerful for me. The sweat lodge became a focus and path that helped guide me towards recovery. I have been participating in drumming circles and sweat lodges for more than twenty years. My local sweat is connected with the Dakota tradition.

Can you find the little girl on the skull? She is being protected by the power of the Medicine Wheel. I feel safe with this power, and it has helped me in my journey away from the sexual abuse and into recovery.

This skull symbolizes the Sacred Buffalo. On its forehead is a Medicine Wheel, which traditionally uses stones to honor the four directions: Spring in the East for new beginnings and exploration; Summer in the South for continuing growth and abundance; Fall in the West for evaluating and making plans; Winter in the North for dreams, introspection, and spirituality. In the center live the Wisdom Keepers, and circling around the outside of the wheel live the Sacred Animals. The little dots are sacred paths.

The Medicine Wheel may be very large, and in a sacred place, some are small and hidden. I had one in my garden for many years. I used special stones my geologist friends collected. It might also be very small on an altar or shelf in your home. It might be hidden in a special bag and laid out on the floor when you work with it. You can use large stones or tiny pebbles or semiprecious stones. You can ask questions to the Wisdom Keepers or the Sacred Animals or the elements. The intent is the important thing.

An idea:

The Buffalo Skull is a traditional ceremonial symbol. Think about creating a symbol of protection for yourself. Both the peace symbol and recycling symbol are inspirational. Can you imagine a symbol for yourself that encourages hope and offers you protection. A circle is a strong beginning. It has the symbolic power to surround and suggest protection. What might live in the center? Perhaps an animal which is majestic or cunning? Perhaps your Power Animal. (Check power animals on the internet to find photos for a medicine wheel you might draw.) Or, you might choose a tree which characterizes strength or a flower suggesting beauty? The sun or moon or waves are eternal symbols. You could draw or cut out the shapes. This project might become a medicine wheel of protection for you. One time, I created a shield using leather and a frame of sticks. I tied the sticks into a tri-angle and attached the leather shield with leather strips. In the center I painted my power animals. These same animals I painted on one of my drums. These two things hold power and protection for me because I made them.

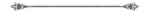

PART III. SCARY PAINTINGS

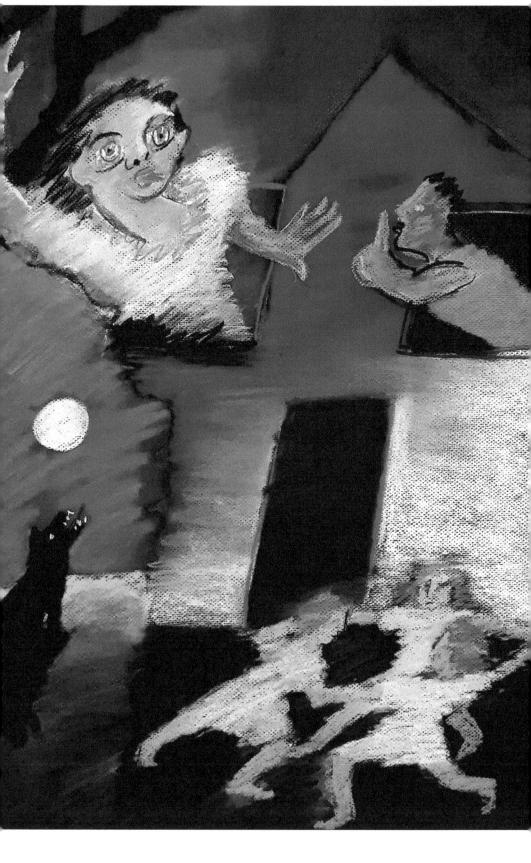

Frightened Girl

The first of the scary paintings is a girl with huge eyes leaning out of an upper window in an old house. Is she about to scream? Someone leans out of the opposite window holding a finger to their mouth, probably saying, "Sh, sh, sh!" trying to stop the girl from screaming. Could that be Mother or Father?

By the time I began my journey searching back into my childhood, both my father and mother had died. There was no way to talk to them. Earlier, when Mother was still alive, she denied anything could have happened when I asked about my being afraid of silly things.

In this painting, the entire house is precarious and looks both threatening and threatened. There are no windows on the ground level. The door has no knob for opening, so no one could come in or go out. The house is incomplete and seems unsafe. My black dog with teeth is howling at the moon—or is he howling for help? There is a sense of frenzy and fear, even in the children's play. Three little girls below are circling wildly. They remind me of the childhood game "Ring Around the Rosie." "Ashes, ashes we all fall down," and we often fell laughing as we sang. This does not look like a laughing time. "London Bridge Is Falling Down" is another song we sang. Those children's songs have hidden meanings of dangerous situations in the past.

Looking at this painting brought back a different tragic memory. While I was growing up, our neighbor was molesting his daughter. I didn't know about it until years later. People didn't talk about things like that. The perpetrator has the power to demand secrecy. Some use threats and some use strange, hurtful games that children trust because there is something they gain like attention they crave or protection for loved ones or they have no power to resist. All the time, the perpetrator has control to command secrecy and silence.

Another memory was of masturbating in bed and replaying my version of Dorothy and the Wizard of Oz. The flying monkeys were very scary and the good witch had to rescue me every time. Then, I could masturbate and feel safe in bed. All of this was my secret.

An idea:

Were there family secrets you were required to keep? Did an adult or sibling tell you never to speak about something frightening, shameful, or wrong that happened? Did you try to tell someone, even family, and they didn't believe you? What did you do? What can you do now? Is there someone else you can talk with? Is there a teacher or neighbor, friend from church or another group, a therapist you can trust? Being isolated is lonely and scary. It takes so much energy to do ordinary simple things when you are afraid. It is as if the world keeps going and you are looking in from the outside. Then it is easy to wonder what is real and what is fantasy. Please talk with a trusted person.

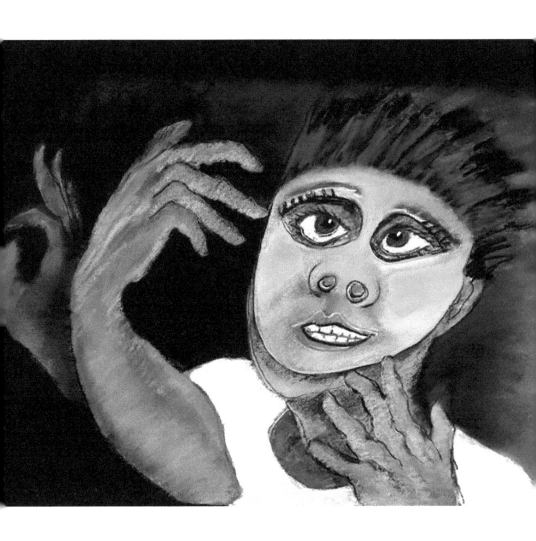

Mask with a Toothy Smile

The mask with the toothy smile is haunting. The nostrils are wide. It is difficult to breathe with a mask and especially when there is tension and fear. Even her hair is standing straight on end. I might know the secret! I might be the child hiding behind the mask? Or, the mask might hide the perpetrator or a family member too frightened to acknowledge what is happening? The eyes seem to be rolling back and up, not wanting to see. This feels related to the time before I started working on my sexual abuse. I did not want to see! At one point my right eye did roll up in my skull and I could not see with that eye. The crooked fingers are creepy, almost like an old lady's fingers, like my fingers now. There is a tragic pleading in this mask. So much is unknown.

On the far left is a shadowy hint of the Buddhist Blessing Hand. Why is it facing away? Perhaps blessings are always available for us, yet we have to be open to receive them, or perhaps the Blessing Hand turns away, not blessing abuse?

Like other symbols, masks can hold numerous meanings at the same time. Masks have an interesting history, from ancient times in Rome and in the Renaissance when masters and slaves exchanged places for a day of crazy celebration. This celebration created confusion with the roles in society. Masks have been important in Africa, China, Oceania, and the Americas. They were used in pageants, ceremonies, rituals, and festivals. They gave power and mystery to the wearers. They can be both beautiful and terribly frightening. Native Americans painted their faces like a mask when they went to war. Masks used during the celebration of Mardi Gras in New Orleans and Veracruz, Mexico, are fantastic. During funerary ceremonies, masks protected the wearer and projected power during a dangerous passage between the worlds of life and death. On some occasions the mask was a shield between cruelty and innocence.

I imagine the mask here is protection to hide behind. It provides a little separation from the "happening." Perhaps this mask protects a child who would like to hide her real feelings behind a crooked smile. Or the mask could hide an adult's plan. When abuse happens in a family, many people want to hide from facts and feelings. Sometimes, it becomes difficult to know what or who to believe or trust.

Masks can hold mixed messages.

An idea:

If you were to make a mask to protect yourself, what would it look like? Would your mask be powerful? cunning? ugly? terrifying? beautiful? You could **draw a mask** *using paint, colored pencils, crayons, or oil pastels. You might* **make a collage** *by cutting out shapes from magazines and glue different eyes and nose and mouth together. (These are simple and quick to make but wonderfully powerful.) On the* **computer**, *within a drawing program, you could create a mask or download images into the program to manipulate. Your* **cell phone** *lets you edit, change, and decorate photos. You can be very creative and no one can see it. There are* **plastic masks for sale** *that can be painted with acrylic paint and decorated with fabric, flowers, ribbons, sequins. Think about a mask that might scare people and protect you. Consider making a mask that is friendly and loving. Sometimes, we forget how loving looks. Who has a loving face? Someone you know, a superhero, perhaps a hero or heroine from history?*

A mask may empower you when you feel helpless, angry, or alone.

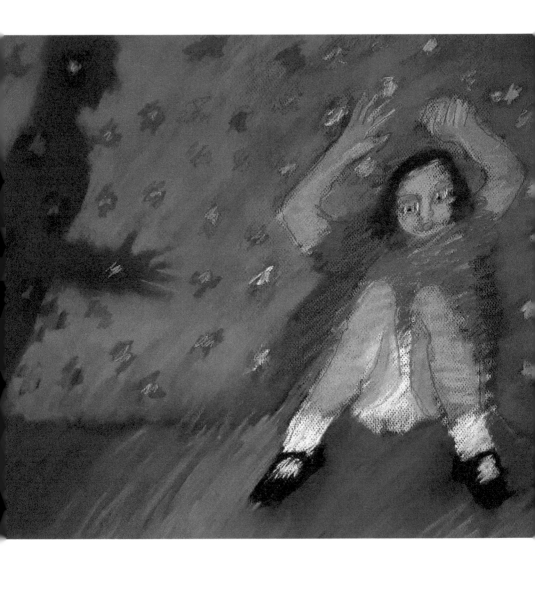

Hiding in the Corner

The little girl is hoping to hide in the corner. She is surrounded by firefly wallpaper. Are they lighting a darkening night? Actually, she cannot really hide. She knows she is already caught because she sees his shadow. She feels helpless, smaller, weaker than the shadowy one. She is too afraid to think clearly, too young to know how to protect herself. All she can do is emotionally separate herself from what happens, from the pain. Denying her emotions may save her in the moment. It is destructive in the long run because in the future she may forget how to identify and feel her own emotions.

The fireflies are an important part of this painting. Like most symbols they can hold many meanings. Long ago on summer evenings, we children used to catch them in a glass jar and watch their lights. Fireflies have filled me with wonder and joy. There are very few now. They have been killed by pesticides. As I look at them in the painting, are they friend or foe? They seem to be swarming like bees, and I am allergic to bees. This wallpaper seems to vibrate and pulse as if alive. Here the fireflies seem to be helping the shadowy one to capture the little girl?

Is it possible to understand what makes mostly normal people become a perpetrator? They obviously have had trouble in their own lives. Caring adults must be willing to believe the children when they tell things that are inappropriate to their age. The truth of abuse is incredibly troubling. It takes so much courage for children to tell their stories. Some perpetrators make frightening threats and some pressure children in other ways to keep the terrible secret.

The children of abuse need support, love, and usually are helped by therapy. The perpetrators need therapy, too. That is not likely to happen unless it is court dictated. Perpetrators I met in jail and prison have a difficult time. Many inmates consider child sex abuse some-times worse than murder.

An idea:

How is your situation different? How do you or did you try to hide? Or was it a game your abuser played with you and then forced you to do things you didn't want to do? Could you try to talk or change the game to protect yourself? Did you have any power? How did you feel about yourself? How did you feel about the abuser? What did you say? What did they say? Do you have power now to protect yourself? It is important to write all that you remember and show it to a safe person. You might need to hide it until it is safe to share. A wise person can help you protect yourself and help release the pain.

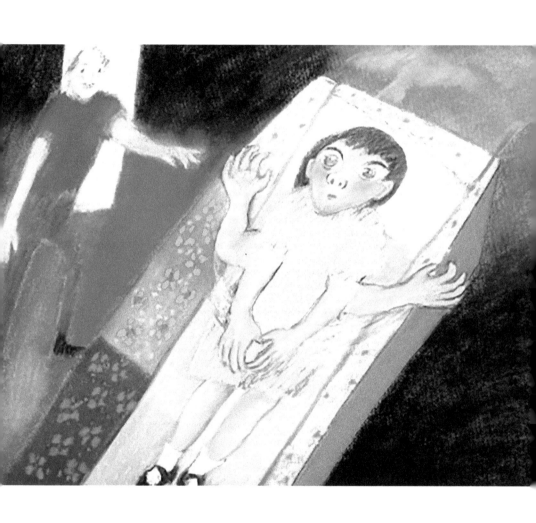

Coffin Bed

Here she is in a bed that looks like an open coffin, still unable to protect herself. Her arms are flailing up and down; she can see and feel, yet her mouth is so tiny that she is unable to scream or even talk. Part of her has died; her innocence is gone!

The coffin bed is a powerful metaphor. She must feel controlled, confined, and almost dead in the coffin bed. It looks as if the fireflies from the previous painting have become flowers that have swarmed like bees into the coffin. Might they comfort her or add to her agony? Now she can really see the shadowy one. It feels like a terrible repeating nightmare.

Sometimes, when life feels so overwhelming, dying becomes a flickering thought.

Please never give up.

An idea:

At one time I considered suicide. I was blessed to have support. There is help available and you can talk with a trained, free counselor 24 hours a day. Dial 1-800-273-TALK (8255). For crisis support in Spanish dial 1-888-628-9454. On July 16, 2022 you will be able to dial or text 988 to talk with a counselor. Thoughts of suicide must be taken seriously.

What is your story? What did you do to feel some control over what was happening? Are you safe now? It is hard to breathe when you are in a panic. Can you talk now? Are you able to eat? Have you lost weight or gained weight? Can you sleep? Do you have recurring nightmares? Do you have frightening daydreams that you can't stop no matter how you try to change them. Sometimes, I felt there was a repeat button on my thoughts and I could not find how to turn it off. The stop button seemed to be missing and it was impossible to use the delete button. Therapy helped.

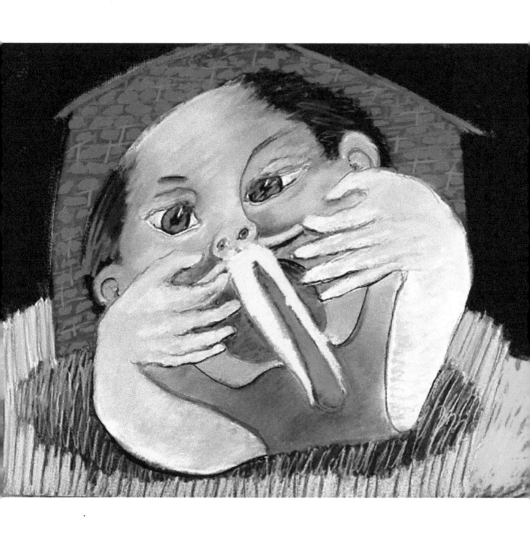

Tongue Looks Like a Penis

The man is holding a doll figure. His tongue is like a penis splitting the little helpless doll. His eyes and hands, everything about this painting is disturbing. Might it be his fantasy, his dream, his plan? The doll is so small, the man has all the strength and control. She has no power to stop him. He might have made terrible threats—to hurt her or hurt her pet or sibling? He might have threatened to tell a made-up story blaming her for everything he made her do.

Behind him is the suggestion of a home. Around the home is a yard circled by a white fence, separating what goes on inside from the outside world. A white picket fence suggests what so many people dream of—a safe, comfortable home—yet so much abuse happens in the home, in hidden places. Abuse can happen anywhere, at any time, in any neighborhood, in any country around the world.

The little doll's eyes are the man's nostrils. Or are his nostrils all she sees? He seems to play with her like a puppet.

He is wearing khaki green, a color which frightens me. It reminds me of the military. Must she follow his orders?

An idea:

Sexual abuse changes how you feel about sex even years later. An adult sexual partner could become the enemy. Abuse changes how you can trust a partner or even a friend. Most important is to trust and respect your own body. Gently, tenderly take care of your body even if you do not yet feel the self-respect everyone deserves. Exercise, sleep, and healthy food are essential. Eat lots of fresh vegetables, fruit, and some protein. Limit fried foods, sweets, and fast foods. Sometimes, people gain weight so they can hide inside a larger body and appear undesirable. Abused people may also use sex in an inappropriate or dangerous way.

Support groups and therapy are important! It is difficult, even frightening to think of joining a support group. Even once in a group, it is important to decide if the group is helping you. I was in a group where the leader was very angry and everyone in the group stayed angry. Anger is only part of the healing. It was not what I needed. To move past anger was my goal. When choosing a support group, it is important to get referrals and trust your gut feelings.

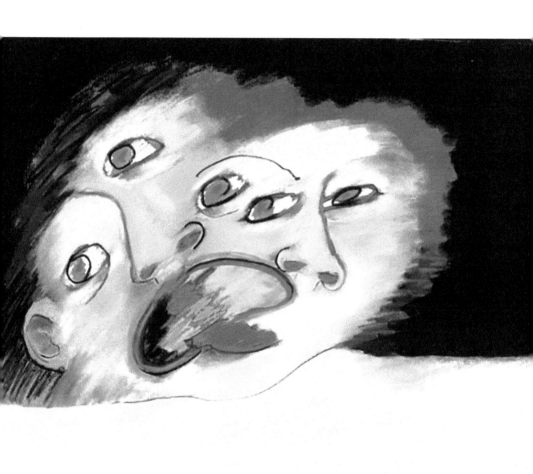

Screaming Face

The screaming face, with five eyes, two noses, and one mouth, pleads for help. Is she screaming? Does anyone hear her? I am not certain she is screaming. Maybe the eyes stare with shock, fear, agony, acknowledgment, and hatred. There are too many different feelings in her head as she slips into mixed-up visions. She cannot focus. It is as if she is falling apart. She senses something bad is happening. Being pinned down with a sheet makes her frantic.

One thin eyebrow tries to bring her many eyes and noses into a single face. A small being is pleading for help and my adult self hears her. I see her nostrils are blood red. In her mouth are blue, orange, black, and green—strange colors to see in her mouth. They do not belong there any more than the red penis tongue belongs there. The larger blue area feels calmer, maybe hopeful? Or is it an open space where she can leave her body and disappear into the unknown?

An idea:

Things happen in abuse that are too terrible to remember. They get hidden. Some people stay angry all their lives without remembering why. The reasons have been hidden in their unconscious mind. People uncover things in the unconscious during creative therapy work, or other creative work like making art, writing, creating music and dancing. Hypnosis is another way to explore the unconscious. Exploration may take time, yet it is worth the effort. Some people find partners, friends, and therapists who can support them as they work through the trauma.

We choose how we live our lives. Living with confusing shock, fear, agony, and hatred can be overwhelming. It is important to identify the details and events that link to these emotions. Acknowledge, respect, and express your feelings, even the ones you are reluctant to face and understand. For example, anger was not allowed in my family so I didn't know how to express it. You have a right to be very angry, yet continuing anger causes more pain and tension that can weaken the body. It can also create a lonely life because people close to you maybe uneasy around constant anger. If possible, do not live with massive anger or ignore overwhelming emotions that are destructive.

Another option is to ask: "What do I need to learn from this situation?" "Who do I need to talk with?" "What can I do to protect myself now?" "How can I trust now after being betrayed?" Search for answers to these questions. It may sound analytical, intuitive, even spiritual, yet these new understandings can open a path to your recovery.

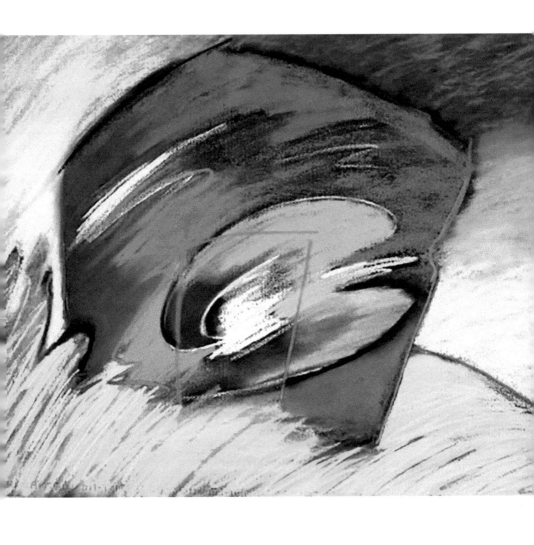

Clam Shell House

Another house, this time inside is the addition of a clam shell. What a strange symbol inside a house. In front of the clam shell, three straight magenta lines suggest a door. It is not a door that could open to allow an escape. It is not an opening that could let a helper inside.

Why is a clam shell in a house? When a clam is closed, it is very difficult to pry open. The victim is tragically caught as if trapped in a clam shell, suffocating and bound to the abuser in silence. It is difficult for the abuser to admit the wrong and seek help. It can feel as if there is no support or way out. Here the shell is open—a positive sign. It seems to be splitting and spitting something out! White scribbles above the shell only hint at windows. They give no way for those outside to see the problem. Those inside remain blind to what is possible. The scribbles also look like closed eyes. If these are closed eyes, it is because seeing what is happening is too painful. The clam shell might also be a mouth with a tongue. This clam shell is similar to the mouth in the previous painting of the screaming face. Both may suggest a scream and a projecting tongue. The fiery orange inside the house feels like heat, energy, fire, anger, pain, hatred. The space behind the house seems empty and isolated. The green and blue colors in front of the house cannot hide what happens inside anymore. This place of hidden and unforgiven pain is now opening.

An idea:

There are four images of houses in this book and many paintings of scenes within a house. Abuse can happen in any secluded place. When it happens in a house, that home becomes isolated, darker than before. It is difficult to breathe in the tense environment of a house with secrets. The first step is to ask for help from outside. Simply asking breaks the bond of secrecy, and brings in light and hopefully caring support.

If this clam shell could talk, what would it say? This question can be asked many different times and get different answers. And, that is good. Is it possible to see change? Yes! Hopefully, growth and well-ness evolve!

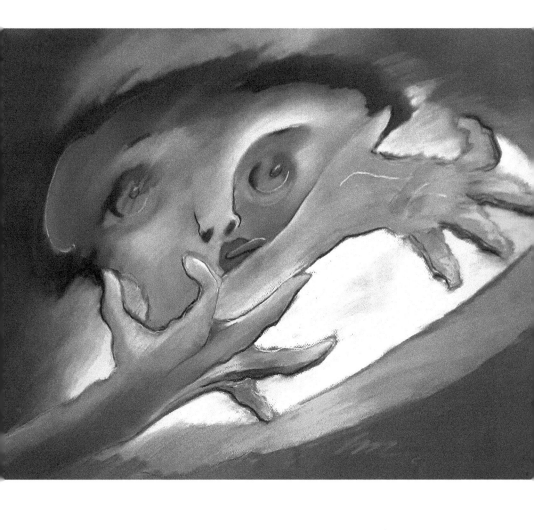

Desperate Pleading

This painting is the most frightening of all for me because it feels so hopeless. Her distorted head feels unconnected. Her eyes seem sunken. One small eyebrow raises a question. Her huge ear is hidden yet listens for anyone or anything coming to help. Her nose looks squished as if she can barely breathe. The fingers are desperately grasping. Are they hers or someone else's? The yellow and greenish diagonal oval swirls around her head, adding to the feeling of being disconnected and unstable. Her tiny tongue is sticking out, defiant. She feels very lost and alone. I see different things at different times. What do you see?

An idea:

I become aware that the ideas and feelings that I express in writing may be different from what other people see and feel when they look at this painting. This is part of the richness of making art, then describing what evolved and what I see in the art at different times. For example, when I looked at this painting after many years, I felt the hands belonged to the face and were pleading for help. Now, I am not even sure they are her hands. This creates a new and different mystery if they are not her hands. This difference in understanding the painting might help you realize how feelings change. Each has value.

Sometimes, we have to reach the very bottom to begin the climb out of our hidden pain and the feeling that our life is broken. This concept of bottoming out is similar to the Alcoholics Anonymous 12-Step program. In the very first step, people acknowledge that their personal lives have become unmanageable. Working the twelve steps is very helpful to see what you can control and what you cannot. Sometimes we need to accept that we cannot solve our problems alone. We need to reach out. Good help may come from many places, sometimes, unexpected places.

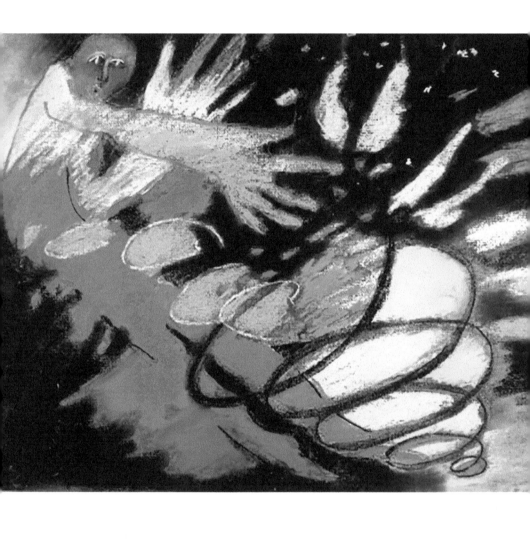

Spiraling Out of Control

Spirals are exploding and splitting from her. She is separating from the terror. Her mouth is in a round "O." Her right arm is extended to guide the release. Her left hand is up, protecting her face as she releases what kept her tied to the past. She is angry! Now with eyes wide open she can see patterns of abuse. She is releasing: memories, nightmares, images, and experiences. This release takes great courage. She is determined to protect herself! Yet, this release is also a sacrifice if it cuts off whole sections of her life. Sometimes, important and good things are lost too. She is losing part of herself in releasing and forgetting. This image came to me unbidden. I don't know what real-life experiences connect to this painting or even if this actually happened to me in this life or another. I expressed my feelings about the abuse by making this art. It allowed me to release these feelings of anger, terror, and loss.

The spiral of this painting is going down into the unconscious. The unconscious is like a personal library or vault where the good and bad are mixed together in a jumble. The unconscious can hold life events, thoughts, and feelings, things we have learned as children. Exploring allows us to see things that have impacted our life without our being aware of it. It is impossible to only access the positive. We must put on our tall boots, gather great personal courage, and prepare for a journey into the dark night of the soul. Travelling this path may not be possible alone. The support of a loyal friend or a group may give light along the path. A therapist can be a partner or guide when wading through a swamp in the unconscious. In this way one can begin to untangle the thread of truth that will set one free.

When I began therapy in my fifties, I was dealing with experiences that happened when I was a baby and young child. In therapy I was not able to recall and examine concrete experiences. I accepted the fact of abuse because of my initial reaction when learning of other abuse in my family. I simply collapsed, became numb, and slumped in a chair. I closed my eyes and decided that this was not going to stop me. I wanted to keep living as if nothing had changed. Yet tears filled my heart until I was faced with a life/death physical problem. My right eye rolled up so that I could not see; only the white of the eye showed. At this time, I could neither teach nor create my own art. My right eye saw what my heart knew, yet still my mind would not see. My eye turned inward. Since doctors could not diagnose what was happening, my college opened an opportunity for me to retire. I was referred to an optical professional who gave me eye exercises which strengthen and greatly corrected my right eye. When I no longer saw double, I started therapy and the search for the truth of my sexual abuse. Intuitively, I knew it was central to my recovery. In therapy, I responded so vehemently to the art I was creating that I accepted its truth. Sometimes I related personally and sometimes on a universal level. I had lived my life with some ghostly images, some of which I now know were literally true and some are still a mystery. Recently, finding the photograph of me as a little girl and analyzing her tragic drawing was another powerful validation of sexual abuse. Accepting the facts and feelings of abuse can be an ongoing healing process. Even recognizing only some of the past abuse has not stopped me from living a meaningful life.

I have learned much and been blessed.

An idea:

I believe that the unconscious also holds information from our past lives, the lives of our parents, and their parents in history. When I was in Sweden, the country, the trees, and the people seemed so familiar, yet I had never been there before. The concept of past lives is important in many religions. I first began thinking about past lives when I was in Japan for three weeks, sightseeing, waiting for my first granddaughter to be born and reading books. Much later, I began using past lives to help me and clients understand what was happening in our lives and why it might feel like déjà vu. Understandings from past lives have also helped me in relationships with some people. There have been places in Japan, India, Sweden, and Mexico that seemed very familiar. DNA validated that as true. This begins to seem plausible with so many people tracing their DNA and learning their past family history.

The reason I mention past lives now is because I believe sexual abuse had happened to me before, in a past life. That is why the images came so vividly and powerfully and my body reacted with strong emotion. I believe that abuse returned so I could clear it forever. That way, I pray, it never will return again.

Do these ideas make sense for you? What places in the world do you want to visit? Where have you felt a connection? Where have you visited for the first time yet it felt very familiar? Have you passed a person in a crowd and felt a connection with them? All of these situations might be indications of past lives. Sometimes I simply honor them and sometimes I use hypnosis to make a connection.

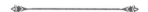

PART IV. CONSCIOUS MEMORIES

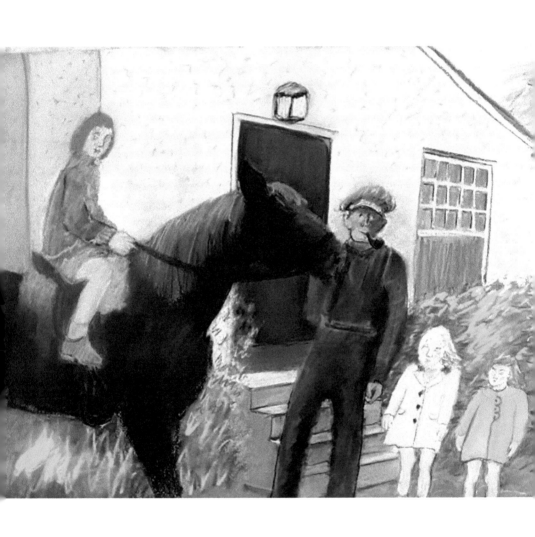

Ann On a Horse

The earlier paintings were pulled from my unconscious or were intuitive gifts. They are not totally my experiences, although they feel true for me. My heart races and my stomach fills with tight knots sometimes when I look at them. I believe they depict, in part, what happened to me as a very young child—so young I do not remember clearly. They depict some of what happened to me in this life and past lives, and some of what happened to others. Yet, when I saw the old photo of my little self on the rocking horse with the drawing I had done on the blackboard, abuse was a reality I could not deny.

I clearly remember this episode of the man with a horse. I was in second grade and we lived in a small northern rural community. One day a man came by our home on a horse driving a herd of goats. It was very exciting to see all the animals herded past our home. The man— I call him The Goat Man—stopped and talked. He saw that I loved horses and he promised to return and take me for a ride. I begged my mother to let me ride if he returned. Because I love horses, I put myself in danger.

Little could I imagine the horror that would follow.

An idea:

Have you ever wanted something very much only to learn that it was not good for you? Sometimes it seems impossible to know that what looks wonderful, is actually dangerous. Do you listen to your heart? How do you learn? Have you ever wanted something very much? Did you go ahead and do it even though it might be dangerous? What did you learn? This is something to journal.

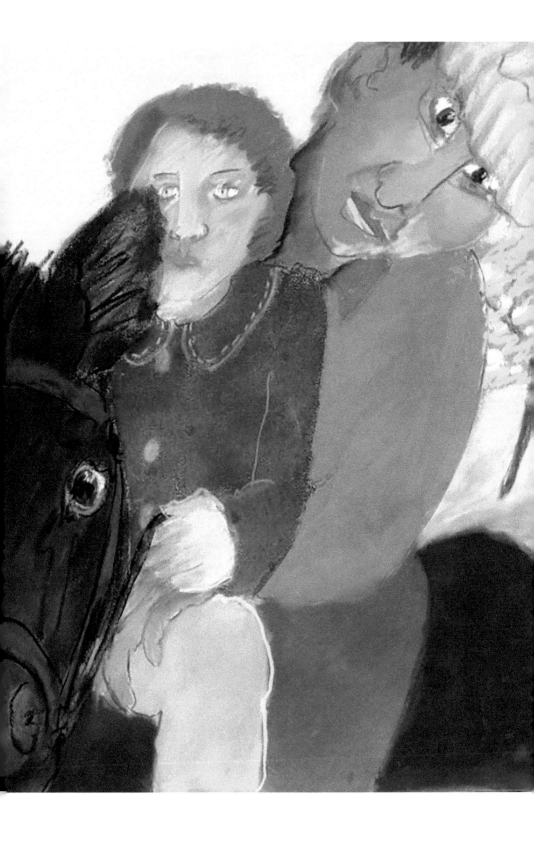

Goat Man's Intentions

The Goat Man did return. The first ride was OK. In fact, it was fun! He came back again, and I was delighted. He was building my young child's trust. On the second ride he took the horse in an unfamiliar direction and I became scared. When he began rubbing my thigh I became paralyzed. I could not jump off the horse and run away. In the painting, it is easy to see the Goat Man's intentions. His fingers are gliding toward my genitals. The horse reacts in horror, while I become frozen, like a statue. Somehow, I got back home—very frightened, yet safe. I never again went for a ride with the Goat Man; in fact, I never saw the Goat Man again.

Later, I did visit horses in our community. I got bitten once when I tried to share my Peppermint Patty with a horse. Instead of licking the paper as dogs do, he bit me. That didn't stop me from visiting that horse and going horseback riding on the special occasions when I earned enough money from babysitting to rent a horse from a reliable stable.

An idea:

Have you ever been hardheaded and determined to do what seems the fun thing to do? How did it evolve? What did you learn? Slowly, I learned that there are things I need to do but it takes time to know the rules. It takes practice and patience to do it well. Hopefully, I am able to evaluate the process and ask for advice when I need it. There are always people who have more experience and are gladly willing to help. That is a lesson I am still learning!

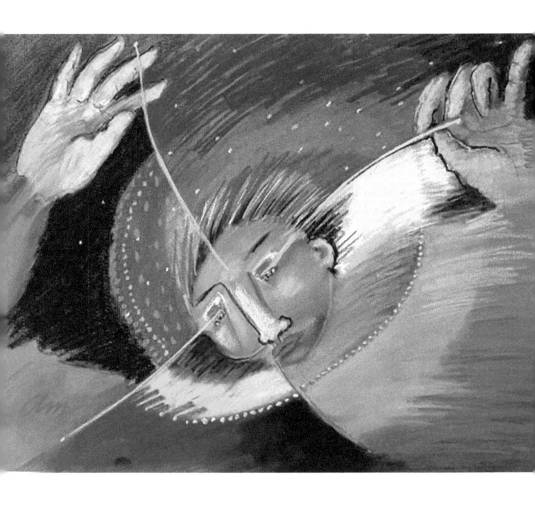

Angel of Protection

This angel comes from the stars to help protect and guide people. I believe we all have angels. They are always there for me when I ask for help. Sometimes the voices of abusers, present or past, make it hard to hear your angels. If other gentle people did not hear you cry or see the trouble, could an angel? Yes! **It is OK to ask for help.** That is a tough lesson.

It is great to be independent, yet learning is a complex process. Healing takes support, time, and good hard work, which may include: individual therapy, group work, dream work, meditation, diaries, writing, painting, singing, dancing, sewing, woodworking, gardening, walking, running, and other activities. Sometimes these activities illuminate the process and sometimes comfort. Sometimes they bring a childlike sense of wonder. Some of these activities provide sacred space or a sense of peace away from the struggle to understand your present, past, and future.

Angels may come to you in any season of the year, any season of your life, or any season of your healing work. The angel in this painting guides me in all seasons, at all times. Her eyes intently focus, seeing clearly to my heart. The hands are blessing as they gently bring the truth into focus. The angel protects without harming others. For your angel to help, you will need to ask, then be open to their presence. Sometimes the answer comes as words ... like seeing a street sign that answers the question. Sometimes, it is an intuitive understanding. It might be like seeing an ad on TV that gives you an idea and an answer. Be open to what happens around you. Answers and angels may come in unique ways with familiar or unfamiliar voices. Ask for help. Be gentle with yourself. It may take practice to discover answers in intuitive ways. Angels may also be people in human form. They may be friends or relatives, teachers, leaders, historical figures, a character in a book. They may come in dreams or real life. Whenever angels appear in your life, you are blessed.

I am close to my angel when I am gardening. I also talk to my plants and they let me know when they need water or loving care. It's a wonderful way to create new life and beauty. My mother gardened, my sisters, my children, and grandchildren garden. Being in nature is calming. Some of us ski, surf, swim, exercise, hike, climb mountains, camp, play in sports, and some sit alone in the woods or a park breathing fresh air and listening to the trees, the birds, the wind, and the grasses. We can all find magic in the clouds that surround us. In nature it is possible to heal and find peace. Although we may not have superpowers, we can ask for help.

Guided by higher wisdom and life in the stars, this angel helps people develop trust and love. Even though we all have angels to guide and protect us, "bad things happen to good people." Sometimes, I don't listen, yet, if I take the time to understand the situation, I learn from the trouble that follows. Because of pain in my life, I am sometimes a control freak. That is not the best or easiest way to learn or hear my angels calling. I am hardheaded and have trouble trusting. Yet, I believe that I was born for dancing, being creative, and loving others. These eighty-five years have been a long learning process and it is worth it! Finally, my journey finds me grown up: old, healthy, happy, creative, spiritual, and content most of the time. I pray all people find trust, peace, and love. I have been blessed.

An idea:

Do you believe in angels? Does religion help? Are there people who are blessings in your life? How can you be a blessing in someone else's life? Small deeds matter! Every smile counts. What makes you laugh? How can you share it? So many people make our life easier, like the people stocking in the grocery store, the checkout clerk, the mail delivery person, the bus driver, the garbage collector. Like angels, all these people are very important to our life and we often do not even notice them and forget to thank them.

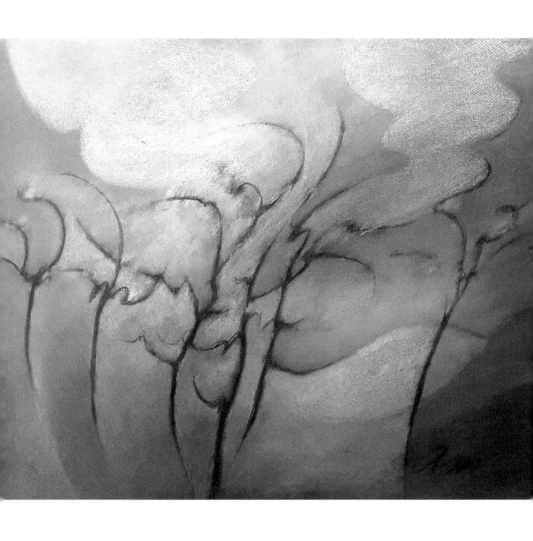

Dancing Dogwood Trees

The dogwood trees are dancing in the fresh spring air. I painted this after my mother died. She loved dogwood trees and I do too. The painting reminds me that I can choose any time as an opportunity for new beginnings, for finding the courage to let go of old baggage. Resolving sexual abuse may take working and reworking the memories. As life keeps happening, new aspects appear. Suddenly there are more feelings and strong images to acknowledge and express. Clearing and releasing is good.

The dogwoods dance and I am reminded that the physical freedom of dance helps release tension and calm my body. Dance is also an important way for me to express emotions like fear and pain. I used unhealthy beliefs about my body like a shield. Thoughts like "I am ugly" and "I don't trust my body because it gets me in trouble." Although those thoughts might have protected me at one time, I do not want or need them now. Zumba dance exercise is my new love because I can release and trust my body in it. Dancing in the group is exhilarating because all my friends are letting go together. We all have things to release.

An idea:

How do you change old patterns and habits? Sometimes just recognizing them helps. Do you have something you are ready to release? The AA program's 12 Steps offer important help in making amends, letting go of baggage, forgiving other people, and especially forgiving yourself. Originally developed by the members of Alcoholics Anonymous, these twelve steps are the foundation for a variety of anonymous self-help groups, including meetings for survivors of sexual abuse. Working on these steps helps people clarify what is and what is not their fault and discover a responsible way forward, free of guilt and shame, respecting themselves and others.

During times of momentous change in our inner lives and our outer lives, the natural world can surround us with gentle beauty and healing power. In those quiet times I pray we can breathe in silence together. The unpredictable, frightening side of nature comes with natural disasters like fires, tornadoes, earthquakes, floods, droughts, tsunamis, volcanoes, and earthquakes. We are reminded again and again that we are not in control. We have abused nature. Native peoples protect and honor all of nature. I have much to learn from them. Their cycles of nature provide opportunities for living with respect in all seasons: spring—new beginnings, summer—time of growth, fall—evaluating the progress, and winter—looking to spiritual power for guidance. Although climate change continues, we have the opportunity to work to protect our earth and live responsibly. We can work toward a loving world. With renewed courage I pray we can move beyond the present confusion into a future where we listen to each other, respect differences and work for compromise, balance and healing.

Epilogue

The pastel paintings in the book speak to the pain and anguish of sexual abuse. They grew from my therapy when words were not enough. People, young and old, healing from abuse and those who care about them may identify with the images and learn from what the visuals teach. My heart goes out to you. It took years for me to recognize that I had been abused, name my abuser, and begin the work of recovery. I knew that I had an oddly tenuous relationship with my father. He was distant and I felt rejected by him. Growing into my teenage body was an uncomfortable time, and dating was beyond difficult. I felt very insecure and didn't trust easily. Looking back in time I could identify a variety of psychological problems, yet sexual abuse was not one of them. Finally, I became convinced that uncovering, untangling, and understanding sexual abuse was important for my overall well-being.

I feel that the images in these pastel paintings may be helpful to children even though many of the images can be scary. Sexual abuse is scary. Sometimes, when it is difficult to find words to describe what happened, images can speak. Talking about the paintings can help some children find their own voice. These pastels may give people permission to create their own expressive art. The art can say "This is how it was for me." With or without words, art can speak.

For many years I worked as a volunteer with Hospice. I visited children who were dying and children who'd lost a parent or sibling. Each time I came to their home they would tell me what was happening, then we would work on the next step and what they needed. Imminent death pushed us to face other truths like the future. There is no hiding from death, it is difficult for everyone. One time when visiting a child whose mother was dying, the child immediately hid in a closet. She needed distance from that terrible truth. So, I sat on the floor and we talked through the closet door. This honored her space and helped her through that day. Death is complex and an awesome adversary; yet, that loss was an ending. Sexual abuse is a different issue in that it is not an ending and needs to be untangled.

I feel sexual abuse is tragic like death, yet more difficult to process. Sexual abuse can be denied, making it harder to face. Working with art is similar to talking through the closet door. The art process has a beginning and an ending like opening and closing a door. Creating is also like the closet door in that the activity provides some separation and space from the fear and rage that accompanies sexual abuse. Creating provides a container for the emotions on paper or with clay; the container is outside the person's physical and emotional body and can hold words on paper or in an object. Art therapy worked for me. Perhaps, it will work for you.

About the Author

I was honored to teach at a community college. Because the art department was small, it gave me the opportunity to teach a wonderful variety of subjects: Drawing, Painting, Design, Art Education, Ancient Art History, and Art Appreciation. I get bored easily so teaching different classes kept me learning in many directions. I loved the challenge of teaching and I had the opportunity to visit some of the countries in the textbooks we studied. I experienced historical places and saw original art and architecture in Mexico, France, Japan, China, Thailand, Greece, Sweden, and India. (The gift of travel was thanks to my husband who worked for the airlines, which permitted travel on standby. Earlier I lived for a short time in France and a year in Mexico.) When I began teaching at the college, I also began working on a second master's degree in Expressive Art Therapy. This background was important when counseling, volunteering with Hospice, and working with students.

During my teaching years I was actively attending various drumming circles and sweat lodges. A sweat lodge is an ancient Spirit-lead native tradition. In a small group sitting around hot coals inside a sweat lodge, we honor Mother Nature and embrace the wisdom of the Ancestors. There are always many prayers during a sweat. Because the experiences are so healing, Native American symbolism slips into some of my paintings. I am deeply interested in ancient cultures and honor Native American beliefs, stories, and powerful traditions.

My travel and study of world religions has opened me to the possibility of reincarnation and past lives. Some images in this book might have come to me from past lives. I feel that the pain and what happened in the past can affect me today. The more I can clear and let go of old energy, the freer, more loving and accepting I can be. Each new situation and challenge I work with, understand, and resolve, the happier and more joyful I am. I continue to do past-life therapy for myself and others.

I now live in rural Southern Indiana with my loving partner and a mischievous, mixed-breed dog found on the side of the road. I have a large garden and private space for painting and reading. Three mornings a week I go to the YMCA. I do water aerobics, work on the exercise machines, and take other classes, including Zoomba. I keep exploring spirituality and healing techniques, and I am blessed with family and friends.

I am happy to share my journey, my ideas, and my hopes with individuals and groups. Contact me: ann.healingjourney@gmail.com and healingjourney123.com

CPSIA information can be obtained
at www.ICGtesting.com
Printed in the USA
BVHW051620231121
622345BV00012B/606